AAOS

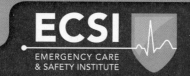
First Aid, CPR, and AED Standard

Sixth Edition

W9-BRB-895

Alton L. Thygerson, EdD, FAWM
Medical Writer

Steven M. Thygerson, PhD, MSPH, CIH
Medical Writer

Benjamin Gulli, MD, FAAOS
Medical Editor

Gina Piazza, DO, FACEP
Medical Editor

American College of
Emergency Physicians®
ADVANCING EMERGENCY CARE

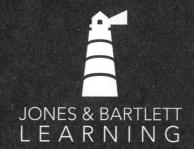

JONES & BARTLETT
LEARNING

World Headquarters
Jones & Bartlett Learning
40 Tall Pine Drive
Sudbury, MA 01776
978-443-5000
info@jblearning.com
www.jblearning.com

Substantial discounts on bulk quantities of Jones & Bartlett Learning publications are available to corporations, professional associations, and other qualified organizations. For details and specific discount information, contact the special sales department at Jones & Bartlett Learning via the above contact information or send an email to specialsales@jblearning.com.

Jones & Bartlett Learning books and products are available through most bookstores and online booksellers. To contact Jones & Bartlett Learning directly, call 800-832-0034, fax 978-443-8000, or visit our website, www.jblearning.com.

Production Credits
Chairman, Board of Directors: Clayton Jones
Chief Executive Officer: Ty Field
President: James Homer
Sr. V.P., Chief Operating Officer: Don W. Jones, Jr.
V.P., Design and Production: Anne Spencer
V.P., Manufacturing and Inventory Control: Therese Connell
V.P., Sales, Public Safety Group: Matthew Maniscalco
Executive Publisher: Kimberly Brophy
Executive Vice President: Lawrence D. Newell
Executive Acquisitions Editor—EMS: Christine Emerton
Director of Sales, Public Safety Group: Patricia Einstein

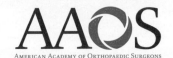
AMERICAN ACADEMY OF ORTHOPAEDIC SURGEONS

Senior Editor: Jennifer Deforge-Kling
Associate Production Editor: Lisa Cerrone
Marketing Manager: Brian Rooney
Composition: Spoke & Wheel
Cover Design: Kristin E. Parker
Photo Research and Permissions Supervisor: Christine Myaskovsky
Photo Shoot Technical Advisor: Bill Kimball, EMT-P
Associate Photo Researcher: Jessica Elias
Cover Image: © Berta A. Daniels, 2010
Printing and Binding: Courier Kendallville
Cover Printing: Courier Kendallville

Library of Congress Cataloging-in-Publication Data

Thygerson, Alton L.
    Standard first aid, CPR, and AED / Alton Thygerson, medical writer ; Benjamin Gulli, medical editor ; Gina Piazza, medical editor ; American College of Emergency Physicians. – 6th ed.
        p. ; cm.
    Includes index.
    At head of title: Emergency Care and Safety Institute, American Academy of Orthopaedic Surgeons.
    Rev. ed of: First aid, CPR, and AED. Standard / Alton Thygerson, medical writer ; Benjamin Gulli, Jon R. Krohmer, medical editor[s]. 5th ed. c2006.
    ISBN 978-1-4496-0944-3 (pbk.)
    1. First aid in illness and injury. 2. CPR (First aid) 3. Automated external defibrillation. I. Gulli, Benjamin. II. Piazza, Gina M. III. Thygerson, Alton L. First aid, CPR, and AED. Standard. IV. American College of Emergency Physicians. V. Emergency Care and Safety Institute. VI. Title.
    [DNLM: 1. First Aid. 2. Cardiopulmonary Resuscitation. 3. Electric Countershock. WA 292]
    RC86.7.T473 2012
    616.02'52–dc22

                                                                                    2010053858

6048
Printed in the United States of America
15   10 9

brief contents

contents

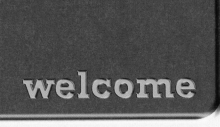

welcome

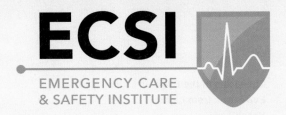

EMERGENCY CARE
& SAFETY INSTITUTE

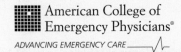

ADVANCING EMERGENCY CARE

Welcome to the Emergency Care and Safety Institute

Welcome to the Emergency Care and Safety Institute (ECSI), brought to you by the American Academy of Orthopaedic Surgeons (AAOS) and the American College of Emergency Physicians (ACEP).

The ECSI is an internationally renowned organization that provides training and certifications that meet job-related requirements as defined by regulatory authorities such as OSHA, The Joint Commission, and state offices of EMS, Education, Transportation, and Health. Our courses are delivered throughout a range of industries and markets worldwide, including colleges and universities, business and industry, government, public safety agencies, hospitals, private training companies, and secondary school systems.

ECSI programs are offered in association with the AAOS and ACEP. AAOS, the world's largest medical organization of musculoskeletal specialists, is known as the original name in EMS publishing with the first EMS textbook ever in 1971, and ACEP is widely recognized as the leading name in all of emergency medicine.

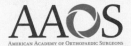

AMERICAN ACADEMY OF ORTHOPAEDIC SURGEONS

About the AAOS

The AAOS provides education and practice management services for orthopaedic surgeons and allied health professionals. The AAOS also serves as an advocate for improved patient care and informs the public about the science of orthopaedics. Founded in 1933, the not-for-profit AAOS has grown from a small organization serving less than 500 members to the world's largest medical organization of musculoskeletal specialists. The AAOS now serves about 24,000 members internationally.

About ACEP

ACEP was founded in 1968 and is the world's oldest and largest emergency medicine specialty organization. Today it represents more than 28,000 members and is the emergency medicine specialty society recognized as the acknowledged leader in emergency medicine.

ECSI Course Catalog

Individuals seeking training from the ECSI can choose from among various traditional classroom-based courses or alternative online courses such as:

- Advanced Cardiac Life Support
- Automated External Defibrillation (AED)
- Bloodborne and Airborne Pathogens
- Babysitter Safety
- Driver Safety
- CPR (Layperson and Health Care Provider Levels)
- Emergency Medical Responder
- First Aid (Multiple Courses Available)
- Oxygen Administration, and more!

The ECSI offers a wide range of textbooks, instructor, and student support materials, and interactive technology, including online courses. ECSI student manuals are the center of an integrated teaching and learning system that offers resources to better support instructors and train students. The instructor supplements provide practical hands-on, time-saving tools like PowerPoint presentations, DVDs, and web-based distance learning resources. Technology resources provide interactive exercises and simulations to help students become prepared for any emergency.

Documents attesting to the ECSI's recognitions of satisfactory course completion will be issued to those who successfully meet the course requirements. Written acknowledgement of a participant's successful course completion is provided in the form of a Course Completion Card, issued by the Emergency Care and Safety Institute.

Visit www.ECSInstitute.org today!

This concise student manual is designed to give laypersons the education and confidence they need to effectively provide emergency care. Features that reinforce and expand on essential information include:

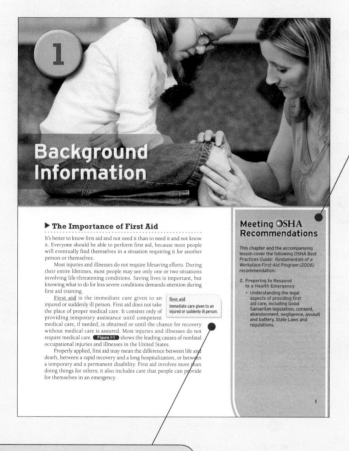

Meeting OSHA Recommendations Boxes Indicate the specific OSHA recommendations covered in the chapter.

Key Terms Key terms are defined in the margins of the chapter to provide students with instant knowledge.

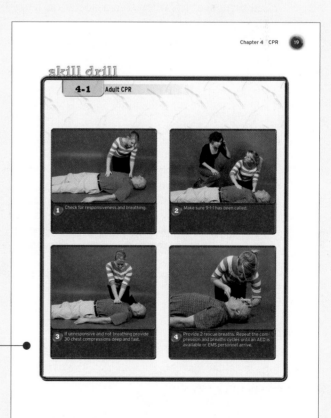

Skill Drills Provide step-by-step explanations and visual summaries of important skills for first aiders.

General Care Guidelines Step-by-step explanations on how to provide care for common emergencies.

Four-Color Illustrations and Photographs Descriptive images and photos enable the student to visualize common signs and treatment options.

Caution Boxes Emphasize crucial actions that first aiders should or should not take while administering treatment.

FYI Boxes Include valuable information related to the injuries or illnesses discussed in that section, including prevention tips and risk factors.

Emergency Care Wrap-Up These decision tables provide a succinct summary of what signs first aiders should look for and what treatment they should provide for the emergencies presented in the text.

---

40   Standard First Aid, CPR, and AED

To care for serious internal bleeding, follow these steps:
1. Call 9-1-1.
2. Care for shock by placing the victim on his or her back and covering the victim to maintain warmth.
3. If vomiting occurs, roll the victim onto his or her side to keep the airway clear.
4. Monitor breathing.

CAUTION

DO NOT give a victim anything to eat or drink. It could cause nausea and vomiting, which could result in aspiration (breathing in foreign material into the lungs). Food or liquids could cause complications if surgery is needed.

▶ **Dressings and Bandages**

dressing
A sterile gauze pad or clean cloth covering placed over an open wound.

First aid kits include dressings and bandages to be used when controlling bleeding and caring for wounds. A **dressing** is a covering that is placed directly over a wound to help absorb blood, prevent infection, and protect the wound from further injury. Dressings come in different shapes, sizes, and types. Dressings can be gauze pads (for example, 2" or 4" square or larger) used to cover larger wounds, or adhesive strips such as Band-Aids, which are dressings combined with a bandage for small cuts or scrapes [Figure 7-6].

bandage
Used to cover a dressing to keep it in place on the wound and to apply pressure to help control bleeding.

A **bandage**, such as a roll of gauze, is often used to cover a dressing to keep it in place on the wound and to apply pressure to help control the bleeding. Like dressings, bandages also come in different shapes, sizes, and material [Figure 7-7]. Elastic bandages can be used to provide support and stability for an extremity or joint and to reduce swelling.

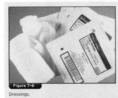
Figure 7-6
Dressings.

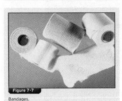
Figure 7-7
Bandages.

FYI

Sutures (Stitches)

If sutures are needed, they should be placed by a physician, usually within 6 to 8 hours of the injury. Suturing wounds allows faster healing, reduces infection, and lessens scarring.

Some wounds do not usually require sutures:

• Wounds in which the skin's cut edges tend to fall together
• Shallow cuts less than 1" long

Rather than close a gaping wound with butterfly bandages, cover the wound with sterile gauze. Closing the wound might trap bacteria inside, resulting in an infection. In most cases, a physician can be reached in time for sutures to be placed. Gaping wounds should be evaluated by a medical professional.

---

84   Standard First Aid, CPR, and AED

▶ **Emergency Care Wrap-Up**

Condition	What to Look For	What to Do
Ingested (swallowed) poisoning	• Abdominal pain and cramping • Nausea or vomiting • Diarrhea • Burns, odor, or stains around and in mouth • Drowsiness or unresponsiveness • Poison container nearby	1. If the victim is responsive, call the poison control center at 1-800-222-1222 and follow the advice given. 2. If the victim is unresponsive, call 9-1-1. Place the victim on his or her side if breathing. If not breathing, start CPR.

Alcohol intoxication	• Alcohol odor on breath or clothing
	• Unsteadiness, staggering
	• Confusion
	• Slurred speech
	• Nausea and vomiting
	• Flushed face
		1. If the victim is responsive:
		  • Check breathing.
		  • Call the poison control center for advice (1-800-222-1222).
		  • If the victim becomes violent, leave area and call 9-1-1.
		2. If the victim is unresponsive and breathing, roll the victim to his or her side (recovery position). Call 9-1-1. If the victim is unresponsive and not breathing, begin CPR.

Drug overdose	• Drowsiness, agitation, anxiety, hyperactivity
	• Change in pupil size
	• Confusion
	• Hallucinations
		1. If the victim is responsive:
		  • Check breathing.
		  • Call the poison control center for advice (1-800-222-1222).
		  • If the victim becomes violent, leave area and call 9-1-1.
		2. If the victim is unresponsive and breathing, roll the victim to his or her side (recovery position). Call 9-1-1. If the victim is unresponsive and not breathing, begin CPR.

Inhaled poisoning	• Headache • Difficult breathing • Chest pain • Nausea and vomiting • Dizziness and vision difficulties • Unresponsiveness	1. Move victim to fresh air. 2. Check responsiveness and breathing and provide care as needed. 3. Call 9-1-1. 4. Try to determine what substance was involved.

Plant (contact) poisoning	• Rash
	• Itching
	• Redness
	• Blisters
	• Swelling
		1. Wash with soap and water.
		2. For mild reaction, use one of these:
		  • 1–2 cups of colloidal oatmeal in bathwater
		  • Calamine lotion
		3. For severe reactions, perform step 2 and seek medical care.

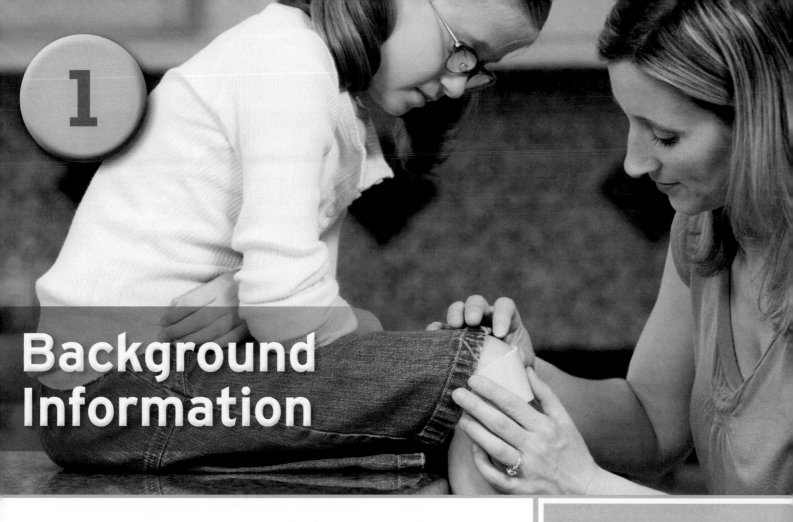

1

Background Information

▶ The Importance of First Aid

It's better to know first aid and not need it than to need it and not know it. Everyone should be able to perform first aid, because most people will eventually find themselves in a situation requiring it for another person or themselves.

Most injuries and illnesses do not require lifesaving efforts. During their entire lifetimes, most people may see only one or two situations involving life-threatening conditions. Saving lives is important, but knowing what to do for less severe conditions demands attention during first aid training.

<u>First aid</u> is the immediate care given to an injured or suddenly ill person. First aid does not take the place of proper medical care. It consists only of providing temporary assistance until competent medical care, if needed, is obtained or until the chance for recovery without medical care is assured. Most injuries and illnesses do not require medical care. **Figure 1-1** shows the leading causes of nonfatal occupational injuries and illnesses in the United States.

> **first aid**
>
> Immediate care given to an injured or suddenly ill person.

Properly applied, first aid may mean the difference between life and death, between a rapid recovery and a long hospitalization, or between a temporary and a permanent disability. First aid involves more than doing things for others; it also includes care that people can provide for themselves in an emergency.

Meeting ⊙SHA Recommendations

This chapter and the accompanying lesson cover the following *OSHA Best Practices Guide: Fundamentals of a Workplace First-Aid Program (2006)* recommendation:

2. Preparing to Respond to a Health Emergency

- Understanding the legal aspects of providing first aid care, including Good Samaritan legislation, consent, abandonment, negligence, assault and battery, State Laws and regulations.

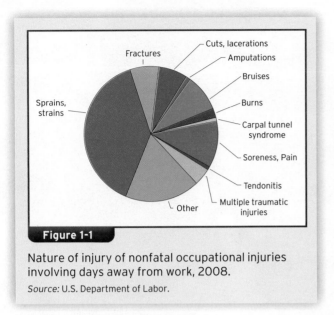

Figure 1-1

Nature of injury of nonfatal occupational injuries involving days away from work, 2008.

Source: U.S. Department of Labor.

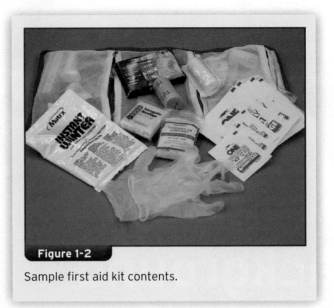

Figure 1-2

Sample first aid kit contents.

▶ First Aid Supplies

The supplies in a first aid kit should be customized to include those items likely to be used on a regular basis **Figure 1-2** . A kit for the home is often different from one for the workplace. A home kit may contain personal medications and a smaller number of items. A work-place kit will need more items (such as bandages) and will not include personal medications. **Table 1-1** lists the basic items that should be stocked in a first aid kit.

Although a first aid kit may have some medications, such as antihistamines and topical ointments, there may be local requirements that restrict the use of these items by first aiders without prior written approval. For example, teachers, activity leaders, and bus drivers in certain areas may not be able to administer these items to children without specific written permission signed by a child's parent or guardian.

The following is a list of medications for specific emergencies that a first aider might assist a victim in taking:

Over-the-counter (nonprescription) medications:
- Aspirin for adults experiencing chest discomfort believed to be associated with heart attack; children and those who are sensitive or allergic should never be given aspirin
- Oral glucose for diabetic emergency
- Antihistamines may help to treat minor allergic reactions

Physician-prescribed medications (the victim must have his or her own prescription to these medications):
- Prescribed inhalers for asthma
- Prescribed nitroglycerin for chest pain
- Epinephrine auto-injector for anaphylaxis (severe allergic reactions)

CAUTION

Note the expiration date on every medication. Replace expired medications.

Keep all medications out of the reach of children.

Read and follow all directions for properly using medications.

▶ First Aid and the Law

Fear of lawsuits has made some people hesitant in becoming involved in emergency situations. First aiders, however, are rarely sued. Following are the legal principles that govern first aid.

Good Samaritan Laws

In most emergencies, you are not legally required to give first aid. To encourage people to assist others needing help, <u>Good Samaritan laws</u>

Good Samaritan laws

Laws that encourage individuals to voluntarily help an injured or suddenly ill person by minimizing the liability for errors made while rendering emergency care in good faith.

Table 1-1 Sample Workplace First Aid Kit

Equipment	Minimum Quantity
Adhesive strip bandages (1″ × 3″)*	20
Triangular bandages* (muslin, 36–40″ × 36–40″ × 52–56″)	4
Sterile eye pads (2⅛″ × 2⅝″)	2
Sterile gauze pads (4″ × 4″)	6
Sterile gauze pads (3″ × 3″)*	6
Sterile gauze pads (2″ × 2″)*	6
Sterile nonstick pads (3″ × 4″)*	6
Sterile trauma pads (5″ × 9″)*	2
Sterile trauma pads (8″× 10″)	1
Sterile conforming roller gauze (2″ width)	3 rolls
Sterile conforming roller gauze (4.5″ width)	3 rolls
Waterproof tape (1″ × 5 yd)	1 roll
Porous adhesive tape (2″ × 5 yd)*	1 roll
Elastic roller bandages (4″ and 6″)	1 each
Antiseptic skin wipes, individually wrapped*	10
Antibiotic ointment, individual packets*	6
Disposable (medical exam) gloves (various sizes)*	2 pairs per size
Mouth-to-barrier device (either a face mask with a one-way valve or a disposable face shield)	1
Disposable instant cold packs	2
Sealable plastic bags (quart size)	2
Padded malleable splint (4″ × 36″)	1
Emergency blanket	1
Scissors	1
Tweezers	1
Hand sanitizer (61% ethyl alcohol)	1 bottle
Biohazard waste bag (3.5-gallon capacity)	2
List of local emergency telephone numbers	1
Mini flashlight and batteries	1
First aid guide*	1

Note: Items with an * sign are required to meet the ANSI/ISEA Z308.1 (2009) minimum standard for a workplace first aid kit. Additional items may be added based on potential hazards.

provide protection against lawsuits. Although laws vary from state to state, Good Samaritan protection generally applies only when the rescuer is:

- Acting during an emergency
- Acting in good faith, which means he or she has good intentions
- Acting without compensation
- Not guilty of malicious misconduct or gross negligence toward the victim (intentionally deviating from established medical guidelines)

Good Samaritan laws are not a substitute for competent first aid or for staying within the scope of your training. To find out about your state's Good Samaritan laws, ask for information at your local library or ask an attorney.

Duty to Act

A **duty to act** requires an individual to provide first aid. No one is required to give first aid when no legal duty exists. Duty to act may apply in the following situations:

- *When employment requires it.* If your employer designates you as responsible for providing first aid to meet Occupational Safety and Health Administration (OSHA) requirements and you are called to an emergency, you are required to provide first aid. Examples of occupations that involve a duty to act include law enforcement officers, park rangers, athletic trainers, lifeguards, and teachers **Figure 1-3**.
- *When a preexisting responsibility exists.* You may have a preexisting relationship with other persons that makes you responsible for them, which means you must give first aid if they need it. For example, a parent has a preexisting responsibility for a child, and a driver for a passenger.

> **duty to act**
> An individual's legal responsibility to provide victim care.

Consent

A first aider must have the **consent** (permission) of a responsive (alert) person before providing care. The victim may give this permission verbally or with a nod of the head (**expressed consent**). Tell the victim your name, that you have first aid training, and what you would like to do to help.

> **consent**
> Permission from a victim to allow the first aider to provide care.
>
> **expressed consent**
> Consent explicitly given by a victim that permits the first aider to provide care.

from a person with similar training in a similar situation. Negligence involves the following:

- Having a duty to act, but either not doing so or doing so incorrectly
- Causing injury and damages
- Exceeding your level of training

▶ Prevention Practices

Prevention practices can reduce deaths, injuries, and sudden illnesses   Table 1-2 . These practices involve three areas of intervention:

- Education
- Enforcement
- Engineering

"An ounce of prevention is worth a pound of cure" is a statement meant to show that it is easier to prevent an injury or illness than it is to treat either one. Prevention requires a combination of interventions that include:

1. Educational or persuasive appeals designed to motivate people to change behaviors that put them at risk.
2. Enforced laws and regulations that require changes in behavior.
3. Engineering changes in products and environment that provide automatic protection from injury.

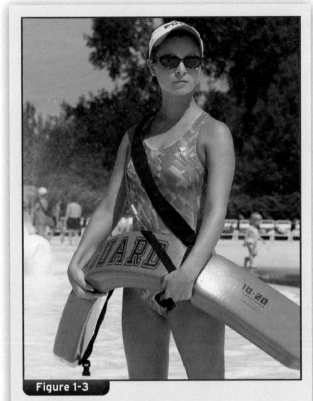

Figure 1-3

Occupations that involve a duty to act include lifeguarding.

When the victim is unresponsive (motionless), an adult who is mentally incompetent, or a child with a life-threatening condition whose parent or legal guardian is not available, first aiders should assume that **implied consent** is given. This assumes that the victim (or parent/guardian) would want care provided.

implied consent
Consent assumed because the victim is unresponsive, mentally incompetent, or underage and has no parent or guardian present.

Abandonment

abandonment
Failure to continue first aid until relieved by someone with the same or higher level of training.

Once you have started first aid, do not leave the victim until another trained person takes over. Leaving the victim without help is known as **abandonment**.

Negligence

negligence
Deviation from the accepted standard of care resulting in further injury to the victim.

Negligence occurs when a victim suffers further injury or harm because the care that was given did not meet the standards expected

Table 1-2 Examples of Interventions

Education/Persuasion
- Swimming lessons
- Gun safety course
- DVD showing safety procedures or messages
- Weather and road condition alerts for drivers

Enforcement/Laws
- Seat belt and helmet requirement laws
- Drunk driving laws
- Prohibiting fireworks
- Personal flotation devices (PFDs) use when boating
- Building codes and inspections

Engineering/Technology
- Air bags in cars
- Helmets
- Child-resistant packaging on medications and chemicals
- Smoke and carbon monoxide detectors

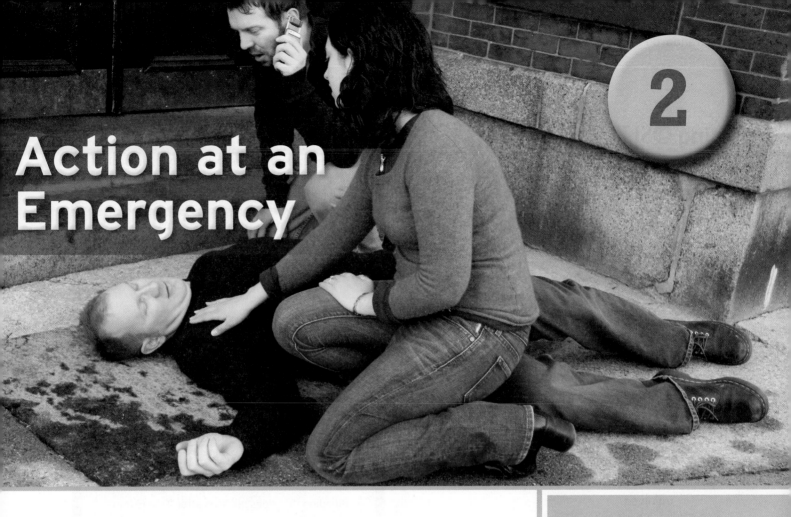

Action at an Emergency

2

▶ Recognizing Emergencies

The bystander is a vital link between medical care and the victim. It is often a bystander who first recognizes a situation as an emergency and acts to help the victim. To help in an emergency, the bystander first has to notice that something is wrong; usually, a person's appearance or behavior or the surroundings suggest that something unusual has happened.

▶ Deciding to Act

At some point, everyone will have to decide whether to help another person. You will be more likely to get involved if you have previously considered the possibility of helping others. The most important time to make the decision to help is before you ever encounter an emergency.

Perform a Scene Size-Up

If you are at the scene of an emergency, take a few seconds to briefly survey the scene, considering three things:

1. *Hazards that could be dangerous to you, the victim(s), or bystanders.* Before approaching the victim(s), scan the area for immediate dangers (such as oncoming traffic, electrical wires, or an assailant). Always ask yourself: Is the scene safe?

Meeting ⊙OSHA Recommendations

This chapter and the accompanying lesson cover the following *OSHA Best Practices Guide: Fundamentals of a Workplace First-Aid Program (2006)*:

2. Preparing to Respond to a Health Emergency

- Interacting with the local EMS system;
- Understanding the effects of stress, fear of infection, panic; how they interfere with performance; and what to do to overcome these barriers to action;
- Learning the importance of universal precautions and body substance isolation to provide protection from bloodborne pathogens and other potential infectious materiels. Learning about personal protective equipment.

(continues on next page)

5

Meeting OSHA Recommendations

3. Assessing the Scene and the Victim(s)
- Assessing the scene for safety, number of injured, and nature of the event;
- Emphasizing early activation of EMS.

5. Responding to Non-Life-Threatening Emergencies
- Wounds
  - Principles of body substance isolation, universal precautions, and use of personal protective equipment.

2. *Impression of what happened.* Is it an injury or illness, and is it severe or minor?
3. *How many people are involved.* There may be more than one victim, so look around and ask about others who might have been involved.

▶ Seeking Medical Care

To know when to seek medical care, you must know the difference between a minor injury or illness and a life-threatening one. For example, upper abdominal pain could be indigestion, ulcers, or an early sign of a heart attack. Wheezing may be related to a person's asthma, for which the person can use his or her prescribed inhaler for quick relief, or it can be a severe, life-threatening allergic reaction to a bee sting.

Not every cut needs stitches, nor does every burn require medical care. However, it is always best to err on the side of caution. When a serious situation occurs, call 9-1-1 *first*. Do not call your doctor, the hospital, or a friend, relative, or neighbor for help before you call 9-1-1. Calling anyone else first only wastes time. Table 2-1 provides guidance on when to call 9-1-1.

Laypersons sometimes make wrong decisions about calling 9-1-1. They may delay calling 9-1-1 or even bypass emergency medical services (EMS) and transport the seriously ill or injured victim to medical care in a private vehicle when an ambulance would have been a better choice for the victim.

Table 2-1 When to Call 9-1-1

If the answer to any of the following questions is yes, or if you are unsure, call 9-1-1 or your local emergency number for help.
- Is the victim's condition life threatening?
- Could the condition get worse and become life threatening on the way to the hospital?
- Does the victim need the skills or equipment of emergency medical technicians or paramedics?
- Would distance or traffic conditions cause a delay in getting to the hospital?
- Could moving the victim cause further injury?
- Do you suspect a spinal injury?

The following are specific serious conditions for which 9-1-1 should be called:
- Fainting or loss of consciousness
- Chest or abdominal pain or pressure
- Sudden dizziness, weakness, or change in vision
- Difficulty breathing or shortness of breath
- Severe or persistent vomiting
- Sudden, severe pain anywhere in the body
- Suicidal or homicidal feelings
- Bleeding that does not stop after 10 to 15 minutes of pressure
- A gaping wound with edges that do not come together
- Problems with movement or sensation following an injury
- Hallucinations and clouding of thoughts
- A stiff neck in association with a fever or a headache
- A bulging or abnormally depressed fontanelle (soft spot) in infants
- Stupor or dazed behavior accompanying a high fever
- Unequal pupil size, loss of consciousness, blindness, staggering, or repeated vomiting after a head injury
- Spinal injuries
- Severe burns
- Poisoning
- Drug overdose

Source: American College of Emergency Physicians.

Calling 9-1-1

To receive emergency assistance in most communities, you simply dial 9-1-1. Check to see if this is true in your community. Emergency telephone numbers are usually listed on the inside front cover of telephone directories. Keep these numbers nearby or on every telephone. Dial "0" (the operator) if you do not know the emergency number. When you call 9-1-1, the dispatcher will request certain information:

1. Your name and number.
2. The victim's location.
3. What happened.
4. Number of persons needing help and any special conditions.
5. Victim's condition.

Do *not* hang up the phone until the dispatcher instructs you to do so. The EMS dispatcher may also tell you what to do until EMS arrives. If you send someone else to call, have the person report back to you so you can be sure the call was made.

▶ Disease Transmission

The risk of acquiring an infectious disease while providing first aid is very low. But it can be even lower if you know how to protect yourself against diseases transmitted by blood and air.

Bloodborne Diseases

bloodborne diseases
Infections transmitted through the blood, such as HIV or hepatitis B virus.

Some diseases are carried by an infected person's blood (**bloodborne diseases**). Contact with infected blood may result in infection by one of several viruses, such as the following:

- Hepatitis B virus
- Hepatitis C virus
- Human immunodeficiency virus

hepatitis
A viral infection of the liver.

Hepatitis is a viral infection of the liver. Hepatitis B virus (HBV) and hepatitis C virus (HCV) infections result in long-term liver conditions and can lead to liver cancer. Each is caused by a different virus. A vaccine is available for HBV but not for HCV. Employers are required to provide free vaccinations for employees who may be at risk for HBV (for example, health care providers).

A person infected with **human immunodeficiency virus (HIV)** can infect others through blood or body fluids. Unless treated, those infected with HIV almost always develop acquired immunodeficiency syndrome (AIDS), which is a major cause of death worldwide. No vaccine is available to prevent HIV infection. The best defense against AIDS is to avoid becoming infected.

human immuno-deficiency virus (HIV)
The virus that causes acquired immunodeficiency syndrome (AIDS).

Airborne Diseases

Diseases transmitted through the air by coughing or sneezing (**airborne diseases**) include **tuberculosis (TB)**. TB has increased in frequency and is receiving much attention. TB, which is caused by a bacteria, usually settles in the lungs and can be fatal. In most cases, a first aider will not know that a victim has TB.

airborne diseases
Infections transmitted through the air, such as tuberculosis.

tuberculosis (TB)
A bacterial disease that usually affects the lungs.

Assume that any person with a cough, especially one who is in a nursing home or a shelter, may have TB. Other symptoms include fatigue, weight loss, chest pain, and coughing up blood. If a surgical mask is available, wear it or wrap a handkerchief over your nose and mouth. Advise the victim to cover his or her mouth when coughing. The victim can be given a surgical mask, if available, if the victim is able to tolerate wearing it.

Protection

In most cases, you can control the risk of exposure to diseases by wearing **personal protective equipment (PPE)** and by following some simple procedures. PPE blocks entry of organisms into the body. The most common type of protection involves wearing disposable medical exam gloves Figure 2-1 . All first aid kits should have several pairs of gloves. Because some rescuers and victims have allergic reactions to latex, latex-free gloves (vinyl or nitrile) should be available.

personal protective equipment (PPE)
Equipment, such as disposable medical exam gloves, used to block the entry of an organism into the body.

Protective eyewear and breathing devices may also be necessary in some emergencies.

Follow standard practices that assume that *all* blood and body fluids are infected. Protect yourself even if blood or body fluids are not visible. At the

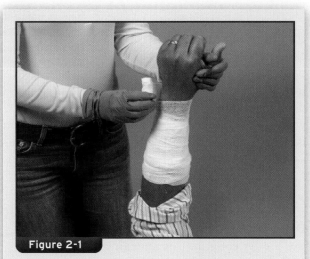

Figure 2-1

Barrier devices, such as medical gloves, are recommended when providing first aid.

workplace, PPE must be accessible, and your employer must provide training to help you choose the right PPE for your work.

First aiders can protect themselves and others against diseases by following these steps:

1. Wear appropriate PPE, such as gloves. If gloves are not available, put your hands in plastic bags for protection.
2. If you have been trained in the correct procedures, use absorbent barriers to soak up blood or other infectious materials.
3. Clean the spill area with an appropriate disinfecting solution, such as diluted bleach (one fourth cup of bleach in a gallon of water).
4. Discard contaminated materials in an appropriate waste disposal container.
5. Wash your hands with soap and water after giving first aid.

6. If the exposure happened at work, report the incident to your supervisor. Otherwise, contact your personal physician or seek emergency care.

Handwashing

Handwashing is an effective way to prevent disease transmission. When washing hands with soap and water:

1. Wet your hands with clean running water and apply soap.
2. Rub hands together to make a lather. Scrub all surfaces for at least 20 seconds.
3. Rinse hands under running water.
4. Dry your hands with a clean towel.

If soap and clean water are not available, use an alcohol-based hand sanitizer to clean your hands.

▶ Rescuer Reactions

After providing care for severe injuries or illnesses, rescuers may feel an emotional letdown. Stressful events can be psychologically overwhelming and may result in a condition known as **posttraumatic stress disorder**. Its symptoms include depression and flashbacks. Discussing your feelings, fears, and reactions within 24 to 72 hours of helping at a traumatic injury scene helps prevent later emotional problems. You could discuss your feelings with a trusted friend, a mental health professional, or a member of the clergy. Quickly bringing out your feelings helps relieve personal anxieties and stress.

posttraumatic stress disorder

A psychological disorder that may occur after a stressful event; symptoms include depression and flashbacks.

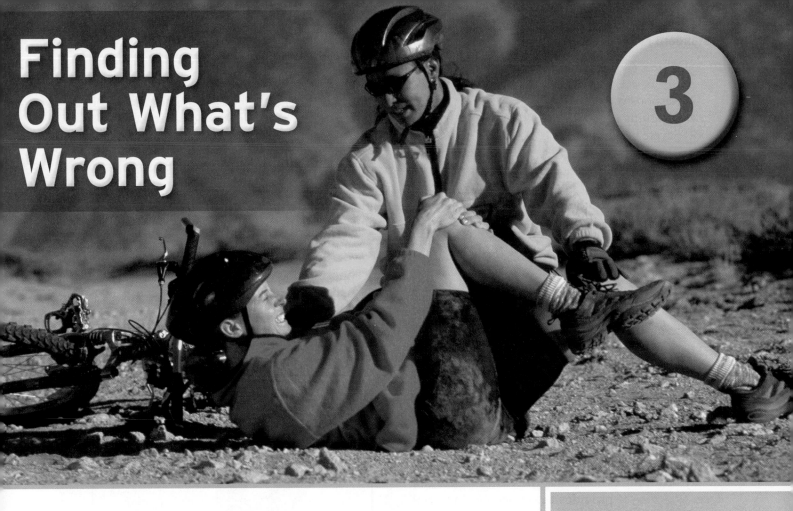

Finding Out What's Wrong

3

▶ Perform a Scene Size-Up

As you approach an emergency scene, do a quick <u>scene size-up</u> to determine safety, the general type of problem (for example, whether it is an injury or illness and whether it is severe or minor), and the number of victims. If there are two or more victims, go to the quiet, motionless victim(s) first. If the scene is unsafe (i.e., downed power lines, fire, or smoke), it may be necessary to simply call 9-1-1 and wait for emergency personnel to make the scene safe. It is critical that you do not rush into an unsafe scene and become a victim.

When you reach the victim, check to see what is wrong. Identify and correct any immediate life-threatening conditions first.

If there are no immediate threats to life, do a quick physical check and gather information (history) about the problem.

> **scene size-up**
> Quick survey of an emergency scene prior to providing care.

▶ Primary Check

The <u>primary check</u> determines whether there are life-threatening problems requiring quick care. It will take only seconds to complete the primary check, unless you find that immediate care is required at any point during the primary check. This step involves checking for the following:

> **primary check**
> The first step in dealing with an emergency situation; this step determines whether there are life-threatening problems requiring quick care.

Meeting ⒪SHA Recommendations

This chapter and the accompanying lesson cover the following *OSHA Best Practices Guide: Fundamentals of a Workplace First-Aid Program* (2006):

3. Assessing the Scene and the Victim(s)

- Assessing the scene for safety, number of victims, and nature of the event;
- Assessing each victim for responsiveness, airway patency (blockage), breathing, circulation, and medical alert tags;
- Taking a victim's history at the scene, including determining the mechanism of injury;
- Performing a logical head-to-toe check for injuries;
- Stressing the need to continuously monitor the victim;
- Emphasizing early activation of EMS.

- Responsiveness
- Breathing
- Severe bleeding

The primary check consists of two steps:

1. Determine if the victim is responsive and breathing **Figure 3-1** .
2. Check for any obvious severe bleeding **Figure 3-2** .

Responsiveness and Breathing

If the victim is alert and talking, then breathing and a heartbeat are present. Ask the victim his or her name and what happened. If the victim responds, then the victim is alert.

If the victim lies motionless, you must determine if the victim is responsive and breathing. Gently tap or shake the victim's shoulder and ask, "Are you okay?" to determine if he or she is responsive. If there is no response, the victim is considered unresponsive.

While checking responsiveness, also check quickly to see if the victim is having any obvious difficulty breathing by looking at the victim's chest and face. **Table 3-1** provides examples of abnormal breathing sounds that you might hear.

Have someone call 9-1-1 for unresponsive victims and those not breathing or having difficulty breathing. Provide CPR for any unresponsive, non-breathing victim.

Severe Bleeding

Check for severe bleeding by quickly scanning for blood up and down the body, for blood-soaked clothing, or for blood collecting on the ground or floor. If you see severe bleeding, control it with pressure.

Positioning the Victim

Properly positioning the victim is an important step in providing first aid. For an unresponsive victim lying face down, roll the victim onto his or her back so that CPR can be started if necessary. If the victim is vomiting, has heavy secretions, or if you must leave an unresponsive victim to call 9-1-1, roll the victim onto his or her side (recovery position) **Figure 3-3** . This position allows the vomit or secretions to drain from the mouth and keep the airway clear. This position is acceptable even if the victim has a possible back or neck injury. If you have additional rescuers, have them

assist in rolling the victim while supporting the head and turning the head with the body.

▶ Secondary Check

With the primary check complete, and no life-threatening conditions present, perform a quick secondary check. The **secondary check** involves a quick physical check for any abnormalities, and gathering information that might be helpful in your immediate care, or for EMS providers if called.

> **secondary check**
> Process of checking the body and gathering information about the victim's condition.

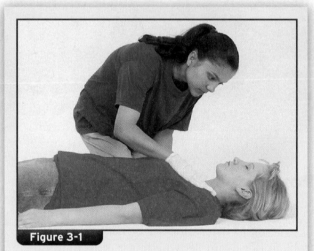
Figure 3-1
Tap, shout, and check for breathing.

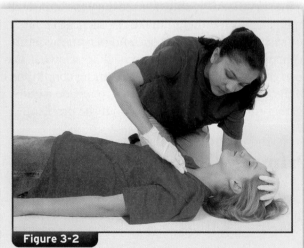
Figure 3-2
Quickly check for any obvious severe bleeding.

Table 3-1 Abnormal Breathing Sounds

Abnormal Sound	Possible Causes
Snoring	Airway partially blocked (usually by tongue)
Gurgling (breaths passing through liquid)	Fluids in throat
Noisy (squeaky or coarse)	Airway partially blocked
Wheezing	Spasm or partial obstruction in air passages in lungs (asthma, emphysema)
Occasional, gasping breaths (known as agonal gasps)	Temporary breathing after the heart has stopped

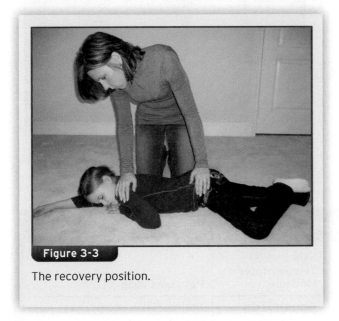

Figure 3-3

The recovery position.

Look for these items during the quick physical check:

- Signs—Conditions of the victim that you can see, feel, hear, or smell, such as seeing a dislocated shoulder
- Symptoms—Things the victim feels and is able to describe, such as chest pain

Most victims do not need a complete physical check, but only an exam of a specific area of the body.

For victims with injuries, look and feel for abnormalities. These include deformities, open wounds, tenderness, and swelling. The mnemonic **DOTS** is helpful for remembering these key signs of a problem.

> **DOTS**
>
> The mnemonic for remembering key signs of a problem: deformities, open wounds, tenderness, and swelling.

- **D** = Deformities: These occur when bones are broken, causing an abnormal shape **Figure 3-4**.
- **O** = Open wounds: These cause a break in the skin and often bleeding **Figure 3-5**.
- **T** = Tenderness: Sensitivity, discomfort, or pain when touched **Figure 3-6**.
- **S** = Swelling: The body's response to injury. Fluids accumulate, so the area looks larger than usual **Figure 3-7**.

Because most victims you encounter will be responsive and able to tell you what is wrong, you can focus your physical exam on the affected area of the body (for example, an injured ankle, painful stomach, or blurry vision).

With victims who have multiple injuries (for example, from a fall from a height or a motorcycle crash), you may have to check the victim's entire body to determine the extent of the injuries. In this case, start at the head and proceed down the body looking for signs of problems. Do not move the victim. To conduct a physical exam for an injury:

1. *Head:* Check for DOTS. Compare the pupils—they should be the same size and react to light. Check the ears and nose for clear or blood-tinged fluid. Check the mouth for objects that could block the airway, such as broken teeth **Figure 3-8**.
2. *Neck:* Check for DOTS. Look for a medical identification necklace **Figure 3-9**.
3. *Chest:* Check for DOTS. Gently squeeze **Figure 3-10**.
4. *Abdomen:* Check for DOTS. Gently push to see if there is tenderness **Figure 3-11**.
5. *Pelvis:* Check for DOTS. Gently push inward on the sides of the hips **Figure 3-12**. If there is any movement, stop pushing.
6. *Extremities:* Check both arms and legs for DOTS **Figure 3-13**.
7. *Back:* If no spinal injury is suspected, turn the victim on his or her side and check for DOTS.

While checking the head, check the color, temperature, and moisture of the skin, which can provide valuable information about the victim. **Table 3-2**

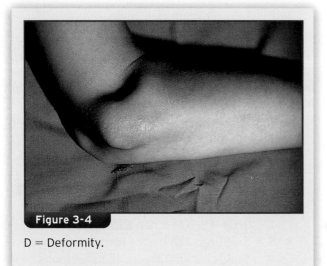

Figure 3-4

D = Deformity.

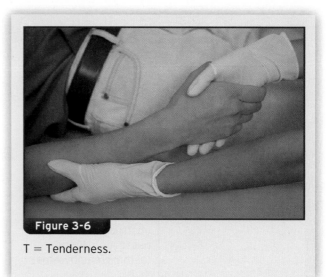

Figure 3-6

T = Tenderness.

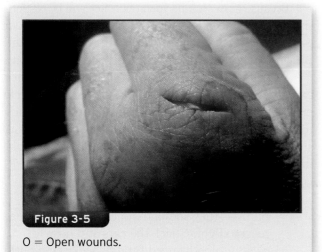

Figure 3-5

O = Open wounds.

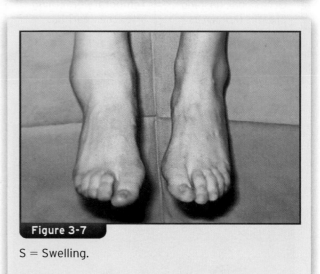

Figure 3-7

S = Swelling.

Table 3-2 Skin Color, Temperature, and Moisture

Skin Color	Possible Cause	Skin Temperature/Moisture	Possible Cause
Pink	Normal color inside lower eyelids, inside lips, and fingernail beds of all races	Warm and dry	Normal
Red (flushed)	Dilated blood vessels from emotional excitement, exposed to heat, high blood pressure, carbon monoxide poisoning	Hot and moist or dry	Excessive body heat (exposed to heat, high fever, heatstroke)
White (pale)	Constricted blood vessels from blood loss, shock, emotional distress	Cool and moist	Poor circulation, shock, blood loss
Blue (cyanotic)	Lack of oxygen in the blood and tissues from breathing or heart problems	Cold and moist or dry	Exposed to cold and losing heat (hypothermia, frostbite)
Yellow (jaundice)	Liver disease or failure		

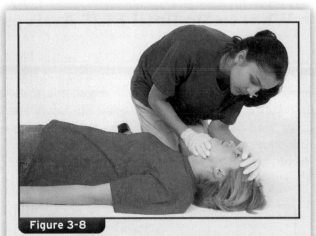

Figure 3-8

Head: Check for DOTS. Compare the pupils. Check the ears and nose for clear or blood-tinged fluid. Check the mouth for objects that could block the airway.

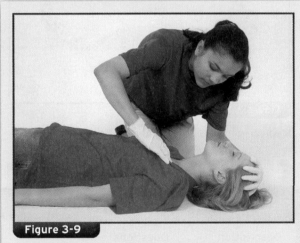

Figure 3-9

Neck: Check for DOTS. Look for a medical identification necklace.

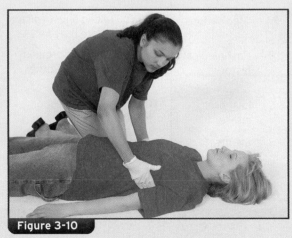

Figure 3-10

Chest: Check for DOTS. Gently squeeze.

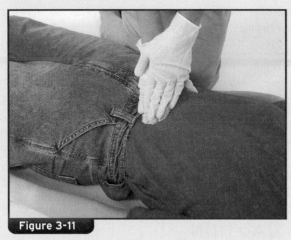

Figure 3-11

Abdomen: Check for DOTS. Gently push.

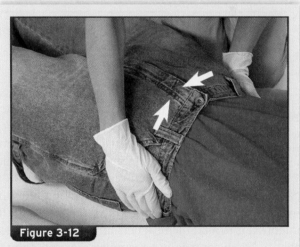

Figure 3-12

Pelvis: Check for DOTS. Gently press inward on the hips.

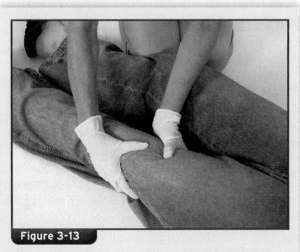

Figure 3-13

Extremities: Check both arms and legs for DOTS.

provides more information on skin color and temperature/moisture.

Low levels of oxygen in the blood result in the skin and mucous membranes becoming blue or gray (known as **cyanosis**). This change is usually obvious in the lips and skin of light-skinned persons. In darkly pigmented persons, it can be seen in the mouth's mucous membranes, nail beds, and inner lining of the eyelids.

> **cyanosis**
> Low levels of oxygen in the blood that result in the skin and mucous membranes becoming blue or gray.

> **CAUTION**
>
> When doing a physical exam:
> DO NOT aggravate injuries.
> DO NOT move a victim with a possible spinal injury.

Medical Identification Tags

> **medical identification tag**
> A bracelet or necklace that notes the wearer's medical problem(s).

The most common type of **medical identification tag** is jewelry (such as a bracelet or neck chain), which provides an inscription indicating an important medical condition that might require immediate medical care **Figure 3-14**. The tag may have a telephone number that can be called for more information. Its intention is to alert medical personnel of the condition even if the wearer is not responsive or old enough to explain.

▶ Gathering Information

> **SAMPLE**
> The mnemonic for remembering key information about a patient's history: symptoms, allergies, medications, past medical history, last oral intake, and events leading up to the injury or illness.

An alert victim may provide information that indicates what is wrong and can indicate the need for first aid. The mnemonic **SAMPLE** helps you remember what information to gather **Table 3-3**. If the victim is unresponsive, you may be able to obtain a history from family, friends, or bystanders. As with the physical exam, gathering this information is secondary if you are dealing with a life-threatening condition.

▶ What to Do Until EMS Arrives

The primary and secondary checks are done quickly so that injuries and illnesses can be identified and appropriate first aid provided. If possible, record information found during this process and provide this information to arriving EMS personnel. Recheck the victim's condition every few minutes until EMS personnel arrive. Record any changes in the victim's condition.

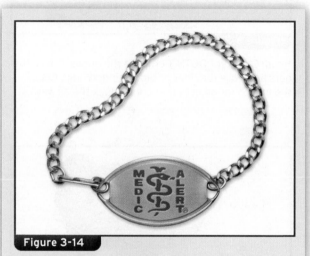

Figure 3-14

Medical identification tag.

Table 3-3 SAMPLE History

Description	Questions
S = Signs/symptoms	"What's wrong?"
A = Allergies	"Are you allergic to anything?"
M = Medications	"Are you taking any medications? What are they for?"
P = Past medical history	"Have you had this problem before? Do you have other medical problems?"
L = Last oral intake	"When did you last eat or drink anything?"
E = Events leading up to injury	Injury: "How did you get hurt?"
	Illness: "What were you doing before the illness started?"

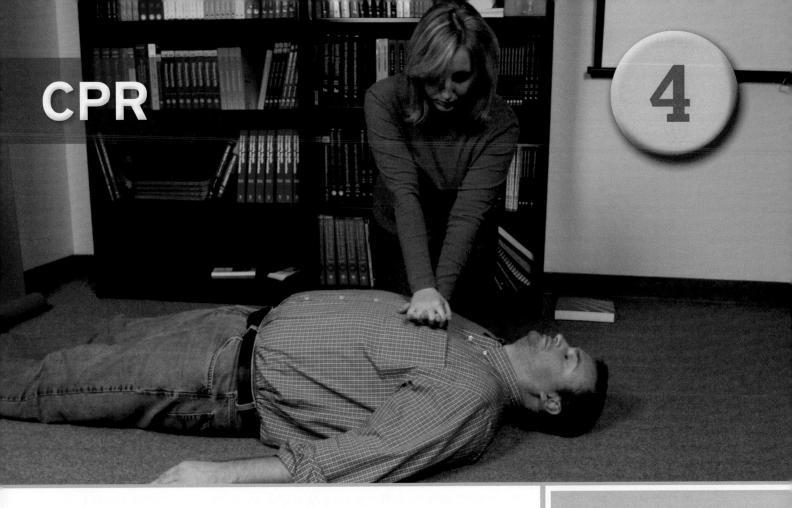

CPR

4

▶ Heart Attack and Cardiac Arrest

A <u>heart attack</u> occurs when heart muscle tissue dies because its blood supply is severely reduced or stopped. This often occurs because of a clot in one or more coronary arteries. The signs of a heart attack and the steps for caring for a heart attack are discussed in detail in Chapter 6.

heart attack
Death of a part of the heart muscle.
cardiac arrest
Stoppage of the heartbeat.

If damage to the heart muscle is too severe, the victim's heart can stop beating—a condition known as <u>cardiac arrest</u>. Sudden cardiac arrest is a leading cause of death in the United States.

▶ Caring for Cardiac Arrest

Few victims experiencing sudden cardiac arrest outside of a hospital survive unless a rapid sequence of events takes place. One way of describing the ideal sequence of care that should take place when a cardiac arrest occurs is to think about the links in a chain. Each link is dependent upon the other for strength and success. In this way, the links form a <u>chain of survival</u>.

chain of survival
A concept involving five critical links to help improve survival from cardiac arrest.

Meeting ◎SHA Recommendations

This chapter and the accompanying lesson cover the following *OSHA Best Practices Guide: Fundamentals of a Workplace First-Aid Program (2006)*:

3. **Assessing the Scene and the Victim(s)**
   - Emphasizing early activation of EMS.
4. **Responding to Life-Threatening Emergencies**
   - Establishing responsiveness;
   - Establishing and maintaining an open and clear airway;
   - Treating airway obstruction in a conscious victim;
   - Performing CPR.

The five events (links) that must occur rapidly and in an integrated manner during cardiac arrest are:

1. *Recognition and Action* Recognizing the early warning signs of cardiac arrest and immediately calling 9-1-1 to activate emergency medical services (EMS).

2. *CPR* The chest compressions delivered during **cardiopulmonary resuscitation (CPR)** circulate blood to the heart and brain. Effective chest compressions are critical to buying time until a defibrillator and EMS personnel are available.

3. *Defibrillation* Administering a shock to the heart can restore the heartbeat in some victims. Time is a critical factor. The earlier the shock, the better the chance of success.

4. *Advanced Care* Paramedics provide advanced cardiac life support to victims of sudden cardiac arrest. This includes providing IV fluids, medications, advanced airway devices, and rapid transportation to the hospital.

5. *Post-Arrest Care* The hospital can provide life-saving medications, surgical procedures, and advanced medical care to enable the victim of sudden cardiac arrest to survive and recover.

> **CPR**
> Cardiopulmonary resuscitation; the act of providing rescue breaths and chest compressions for a victim in cardiac arrest.

FYI

Risk Factors of Cardiovascular Disease

Several factors contribute to an increased risk of developing heart disease. Risk factors you cannot change are as follows:

- **Tobacco smoking:** Smokers have a two to four times greater chance of developing heart disease than nonsmokers.
- **High blood pressure:** This condition increases the heart's workload.
- **High cholesterol:** Too much cholesterol can cause a buildup in the walls of the arteries.
- **Diabetes:** This condition affects blood cholesterol and triglyceride levels.
- **Overweight and obesity:** Excess body fat, especially around the waist, increases the likelihood of developing heart disease. Being overweight affects blood pressure and cholesterol and places an added strain on the heart.

▶ Performing CPR

When a victim's heart stops beating, he or she needs CPR, defibrillation, and EMS professionals quickly. CPR consists of moving blood to the heart and brain by giving **chest compressions**, and providing periodic breaths to place oxygen into the victim's lungs. CPR techniques are similar for infants (birth to 1 year), children (ages 1–8), and adults (age 8 and older), with just slight variations based on the size of the victim.

> **chest compressions**
> Depressing the chest and allowing it to return to its normal position as part of CPR.

Check for Responsiveness and Breathing

In a motionless victim, check for responsiveness by tapping the victim's shoulder and asking if he or she is okay. If the victim does not respond, he or she is said to be unresponsive.

At the same time you check for responsiveness, you should look at the victim to see if he or she is breathing. If the victim is not breathing or only gasping, EMS professionals are needed. Ask a bystander to call 9-1-1. If you are alone with an adult victim and a phone is nearby, call 9-1-1 yourself. If you are alone with a child or infant, give CPR for 2 minutes; then call 9-1-1.

Give Chest Compressions

Chest compressions are the most important step in CPR. Perform chest compressions with two hands for an adult, one or two hands for a child, and two fingers for an infant. Effective compressions require rescuers to push hard and push fast. The chest of an adult should be compressed at least 2 inches; the chest of a child about 2 inches; and the chest of an infant about 1½ inches. The desired position for chest compressions is in the center of the chest **Figure 4-1**.

Give compressions at a rate of at least 100 compressions per minute for adults, children, and infants. Give

---

FYI

Compression Only CPR

If you are ever unable or unwilling to provide rescue breaths during adult CPR for any reason, call 9-1-1 and provide continuous chest compressions for as long as you can (until EMS personnel arrive, you are relieved by another person, or you are too tired to continue).

30 compressions in about 18 seconds and then give 2 rescue breaths. Continue CPR until an AED becomes available, the victim shows signs of life, EMS personnel take over, or you are too tired to continue. Interruptions in compressions should be kept to a minimum.

Give Rescue Breaths

Tilt the victim's head back and lift the chin to open the airway **Figure 4-2** . With the airway open, pinch the victim's nose and make a tight seal over the victim's mouth with your mouth. Give one breath lasting 1 second, take a normal breath for yourself, and then give the victim another breath lasting 1 second. Each rescue breath should make the victim's chest rise. If

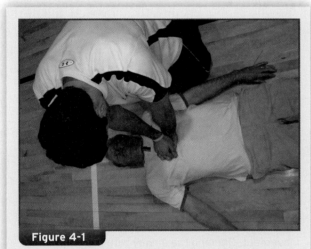

Figure 4-1

The position for chest compressions is in the center of the chest.

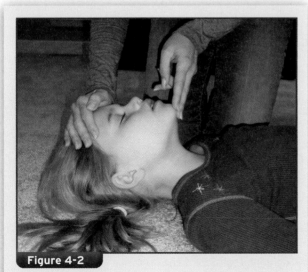

Figure 4-2

Tilt the victim's head back and lift the chin to open the airway.

your breath does not go in, retilt the head and try again. If still unsuccessful, provide 30 chest compressions, look in the mouth, remove any visible object, and reattempt breaths.

Adult CPR

To perform adult CPR, follow the steps in **Skill Drill 4-1** .

Child CPR

To perform CPR on a child, follow the steps in **Skill Drill 4-2** .

Rescue Breaths

Other methods of rescue breathing are as follows:
- Mouth-to-breathing device
- Mouth-to-nose method
- Mouth-to-stoma method

Mouth-to-Breathing Device
A breathing device is placed in the victim's mouth or over the victim's mouth and nose as a precaution against disease transmission. There are several different types of barrier devices **Figure 4-3** .

Mouth-to-Nose Method
If you cannot open the victim's mouth, the victim's mouth is severely injured, or you cannot make a good seal with the victim's mouth (for example, because there are no teeth), use the mouth-to-nose method. With the head tilted back, push up on the victim's chin to close the mouth. Make a seal with your mouth over the victim's nose and provide rescue breaths.

Mouth-to-Stoma Method
Some diseases of the vocal cords may result in surgical removal of the larynx. People who have this surgery breathe through a small permanent opening in the neck called a stoma. To perform mouth-to-stoma breathing, close the victim's mouth and nose and breathe through the opening in the neck.

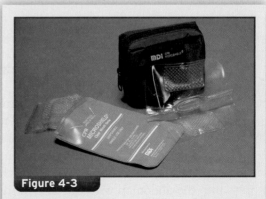

Figure 4-3

Breathing devices.

Infant CPR

To perform CPR on an infant, follow the steps in `Skill Drill 4-3`.

▶ Airway Obstruction

People can choke on all kinds of objects. Foods such as candy, peanuts, and grapes are major offenders because of their shapes and consistencies. Nonfood choking deaths are often caused by balloons, balls and marbles, toys, and coins inhaled by children and infants.

Recognizing Airway Obstruction

An object lodged in the airway can cause a mild or severe <u>airway obstruction</u>. In a mild airway obstruction, good air exchange is present. The victim is able to make forceful coughing efforts in an attempt to relieve the obstruction. The victim should be encouraged to cough.

> **airway obstruction**
> A blockage, often the result of a foreign body, in which air flow to the lungs is reduced or completely blocked.

A victim with a severe airway obstruction will have poor air exchange. The signs of a severe airway obstruction include the following:

- Breathing becoming more difficult
- Weak and ineffective cough
- Inability to speak or breathe
- Skin, fingernail beds, and the inside of the mouth appear bluish gray (indicating cyanosis)

Choking victims may clutch their necks to communicate that they are choking `Figure 4-4`. This motion is known as the universal distress signal for choking. The victim becomes panicked and desperate.

Caring for Airway Obstruction

For a responsive adult or child with a severe airway obstruction, ask the victim "Are you choking?" If the victim is unable to respond, but nods yes, provide care for the victim. Move behind the victim and reach around the victim's waist with both arms. Place a fist with the thumb side against the victim's abdomen, just above the navel. Grasp the fist with your other hand and press into the abdomen with quick inward and upward thrusts (Heimlich maneuver). Continue thrusts until the object is removed or the victim becomes unresponsive. (see *Give Rescue Breaths* section).

For a responsive infant with a severe airway obstruction, give back blows and chest compressions instead of abdominal thrusts to relieve the obstruction. Support the infant's head and neck and lay the infant face down on your forearm, then lower your arm to your leg. Give five back blows between the infant's shoulder blades with the heel of your hand. While supporting the back of the infant's head, roll the infant face up and give five chest compressions with two fingers on the infant's sternum in the same location used for CPR. Repeat these steps until the object is removed or the infant becomes unresponsive.

To relieve airway obstruction in a responsive adult or child who cannot speak, breathe, or cough, follow the steps in `Skill Drill 4-4`.

To relieve airway obstruction in a responsive infant who cannot cry, breathe, or cough, follow the steps in `Skill Drill 4-5`.

> **FYI**
>
> **The Tongue and Airway Obstruction**
>
> Airway obstruction in an unresponsive victim lying on his or her back is usually the result of the tongue relaxing in the back of the mouth, restricting air movement. Opening the airway with the head tilt–chin lift method may be all that is needed to correct this problem.

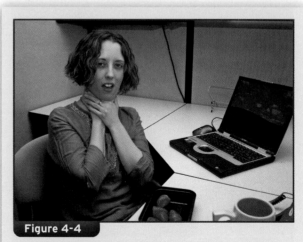
Figure 4-4
The universal sign of choking.

skill drill

4-1 Adult CPR

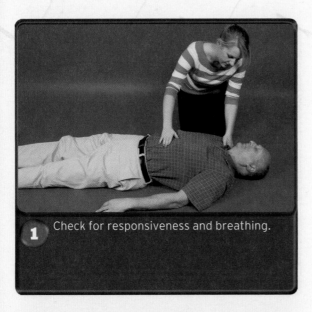

1 Check for responsiveness and breathing.

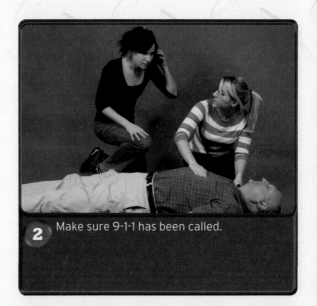

2 Make sure 9-1-1 has been called.

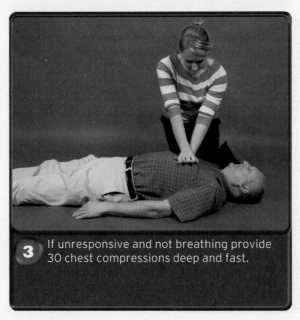

3 If unresponsive and not breathing provide 30 chest compressions deep and fast.

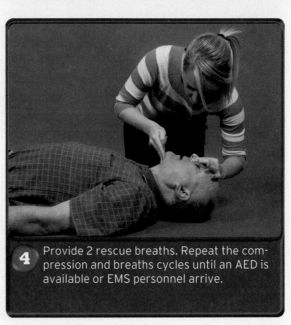

4 Provide 2 rescue breaths. Repeat the compression and breaths cycles until an AED is available or EMS personnel arrive.

skill drill

4-2   **Child CPR**

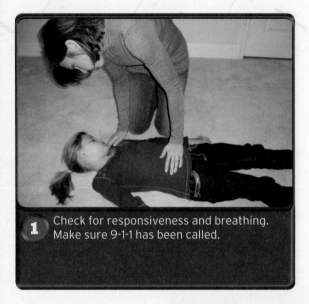

1 Check for responsiveness and breathing. Make sure 9-1-1 has been called.

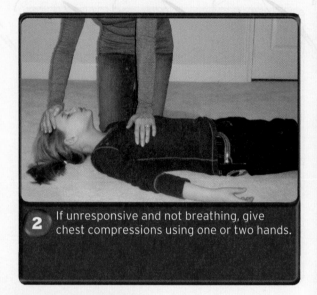

2 If unresponsive and not breathing, give chest compressions using one or two hands.

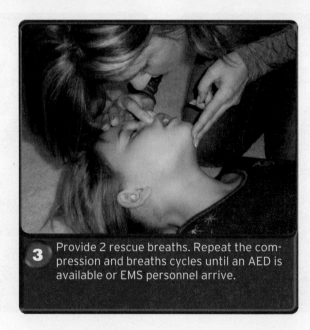

3 Provide 2 rescue breaths. Repeat the compression and breaths cycles until an AED is available or EMS personnel arrive.

skill drill

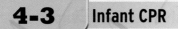

4-3 Infant CPR

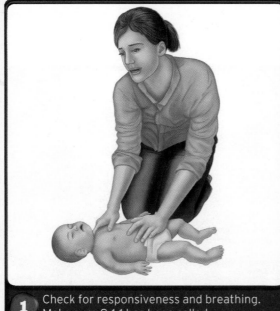

1 Check for responsiveness and breathing. Make sure 9-1-1 has been called.

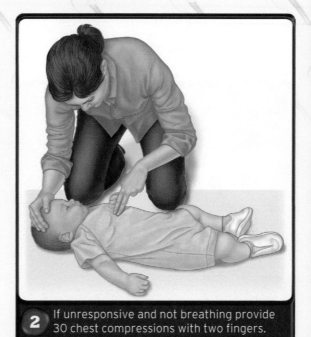

2 If unresponsive and not breathing provide 30 chest compressions with two fingers.

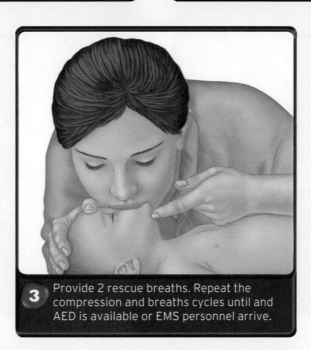

3 Provide 2 rescue breaths. Repeat the compression and breaths cycles until and AED is available or EMS personnel arrive.

skill drill

4-4   Airway Obstruction in a Responsive Adult or Child

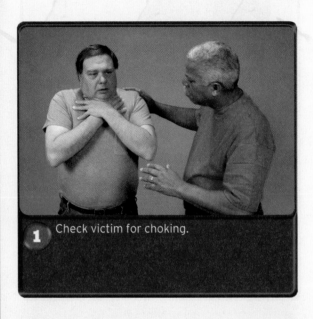

1 Check victim for choking.

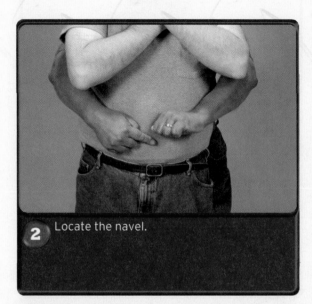

2 Locate the navel.

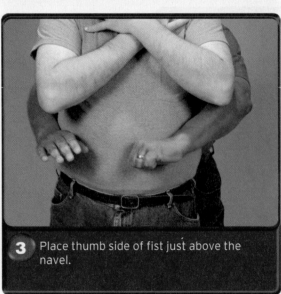

3 Place thumb side of fist just above the navel.

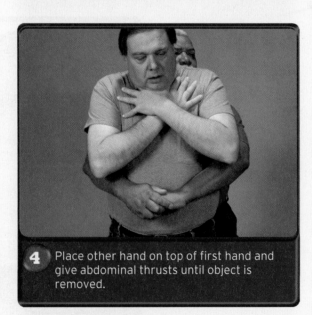

4 Place other hand on top of first hand and give abdominal thrusts until object is removed.

skill drill

4-5   Airway Obstruction in a Responsive Infant

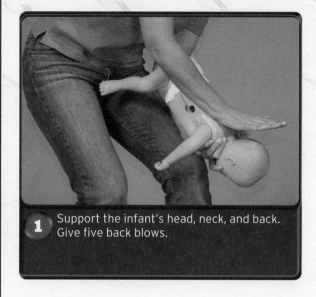

1 Support the infant's head, neck, and back. Give five back blows.

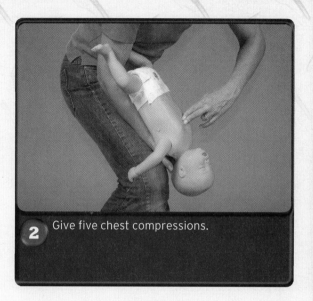

2 Give five chest compressions.

CPR and Airway Obstruction Review

CPR
These steps are the same for all victims regardless of age:
1. Check for responsiveness and look at the chest for signs of breathing.
   - If the victim is unresponsive and has normal breathing, place the victim in the recovery position, and have someone call 9-1-1.
   - If the victim is unresponsive and has abnormal breathing (not breathing or only gasping), have someone call 9-1-1, and retrieve an AED if available. Perform Steps 2 through 5.
2. Provide chest compressions:
   - Give 30 chest compressions in the center of the victim's chest.
3. Open the airway:
   - Tilt the victim's head back and lift the chin.
4. Give 2 breaths:
   - Each breath lasts 1 second to produce visible chest rise.
5. Continue CPR until an AED is available, EMS personnel take over, or the victim starts to move.

Airway Obstruction
For responsive adults and children (anyone over age 1):
1. Check for choking.
2. Provide abdominal thrusts (Heimlich maneuver).

For responsive infants (Birth to 1 year):
1. Support the infant's head, neck and back.
2. Alternate five back blows followed by five chest compressions repeatedly.

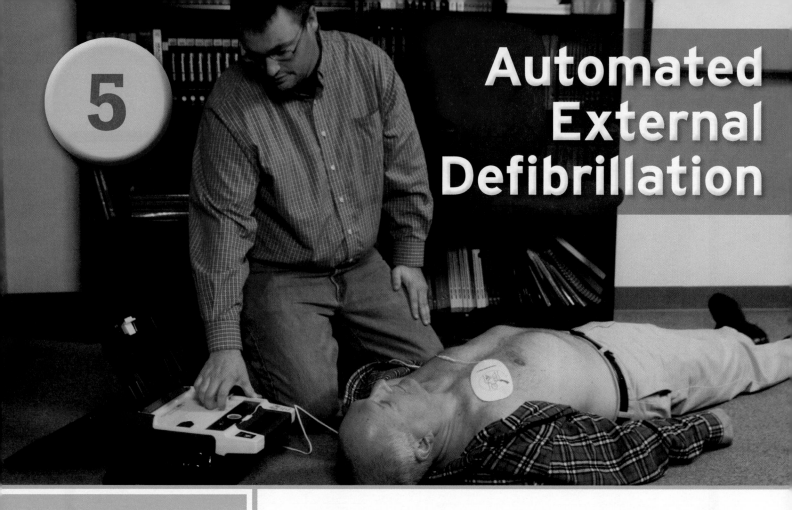

5

Automated External Defibrillation

Meeting OSHA Recommendations

This chapter and the accompanying lesson cover the following *OSHA Best Practices Guide: Fundamentals of a Workplace First-Aid Program (2006)*:

4. **Responding to Life-Threatening Emergencies**
   - Using an AED.

▶ Public Access Defibrillation

defibrillation
The electrical shock administered by an AED to reestablish a normal heart rhythm.

automated external defibrillator (AED)
Device capable of analyzing the heart rhythm and providing a shock.

A victim's chance of survival dramatically improves through early cardiopulmonary resuscitation (CPR) and early **defibrillation** with the use of an **automated external defibrillator (AED)**. To be effective, defibrillation must be used in the first few minutes following cardiac arrest. The implementation of state public access defibrillation (PAD) laws and the Food and Drug Administration's (FDA) approval of "home use" AEDs have made this important care step available to many rescuers in many places, including the following **Figure 5-1**:

- Airports and airplanes
- Stadiums
- Health clubs
- Golf courses
- Schools
- Government buildings
- Offices
- Homes
- Shopping centers/malls

24

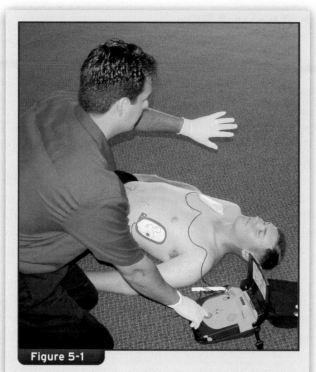

Figure 5-1

AEDs are available in many places for use by trained rescuers.

▶ How the Heart Works

The heart is an organ with four hollow chambers. The two chambers on the right side receive blood from the body and send it to the lungs for oxygen. The two chambers on the left side of the heart receive freshly oxygenated blood from the lungs and send it back out to the body **Figure 5-2** .

The heart has a unique electrical system that controls the rate at which the heart beats and the amount of work the heart performs. In the right upper chamber of the heart, there is a collection of special pacemaker cells. These cells emit electrical impulses about 60 to 100 times a minute that cause the other heart muscle cells to contract in a coordinated manner.

Because the heart contracts approximately every second, it needs an abundant supply of oxygen, which it gets through the coronary arteries. These arteries run along the outside of the heart muscle and branch into smaller vessels. These arteries sometimes become diseased (atherosclerosis), resulting in a lack of oxygen to the pacemaker cells, which can cause abnormal electrical activity in the heart.

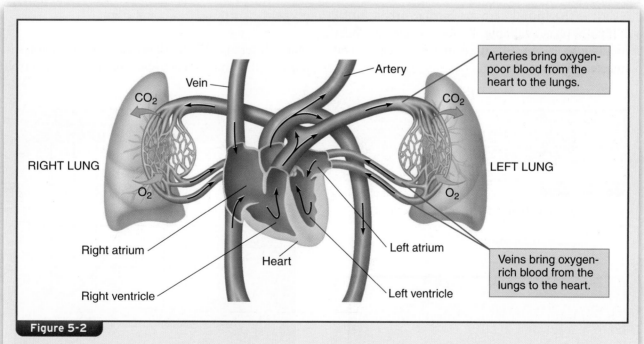

Vein

Artery

Arteries bring oxygen-poor blood from the heart to the lungs.

CO_2 CO_2

RIGHT LUNG   LEFT LUNG

O_2 O_2

Right atrium

Left atrium

Heart

Veins bring oxygen-rich blood from the lungs to the heart.

Right ventricle

Left ventricle

Figure 5-2

The right side of the heart receives blood from the body and sends it to the lungs. The left side of the heart receives the oxygenated blood and sends it to the body.

When Normal Electrical Activity Is Interrupted

Ventricular fibrillation (also known as *V-fib*) is the most common abnormal heart rhythm in cases of sudden cardiac arrest in adults **Figure 5-3**.

The organized wave of electrical impulses that cause the heart muscle to contract and relax in a regular fashion is lost when the heart is in ventricular fibrillation. As a result, the lower chambers of the heart quiver and cannot pump blood, so circulation is lost (no pulse).

A second, potentially life-threatening, electrical problem is ventricular tachycardia (*V-tach*), in which the heart beats too fast to pump blood effectively **Figure 5-4**.

▶ Care for Cardiac Arrest

When the heart stops beating, the blood stops circulating, cutting off all oxygen and nourishment to the entire body. In this situation, time is a crucial factor. For every minute that defibrillation is delayed, the victim's chance of survival decreases by 7% to 10% **Figure 5-5**.

CPR is the initial care for cardiac arrest, until a defibrillator is available. Perform cycles of chest compressions and breaths until an AED is ready to be connected to the victim.

▶ About AEDs

An AED is an electronic device that analyzes the heart rhythm and if necessary delivers an electric shock, known as defibrillation, to the heart of a person in cardiac arrest. The purpose of this shock is to correct one of the abnormal electrical disturbances previously discussed and to reestablish a heart rhythm that will result in normal electrical and pumping function.

All AEDs are attached to the victim by a cable connected to two adhesive pads (electrodes) placed on the victim's chest. The pad and cable system sends the electrical signal from the heart into the device for analysis and delivers the electric shock to the victim when needed **Figure 5-6**.

AEDs have built-in rhythm analysis systems that determine whether the victim needs a shock. This system enables first aiders and other rescuers to deliver early defibrillation with only minimal training.

AEDs also record the victim's heart rhythm (known as an electrocardiogram, or ECG), shock data, and other information about the device's performance (for example, the date, time, and number of shocks supplied) **Figure 5-7**.

Common Elements of AEDs

Many different AED models exist. The principles for use are the same for each, but the displays, controls,

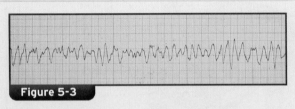

Figure 5-3
Ventricular fibrillation is disorganized electrical activity.

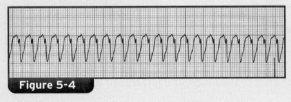

Figure 5-4
Ventricular tachycardia is very rapid electrical activity.

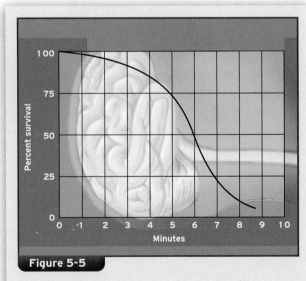

Figure 5-5
A victim's chance of survival decreases with every minute that passes without proper care.

and options vary slightly. You will need to know how to use your specific AED. All AEDs have the following elements in common:

- Power on/off mechanism
- Cable and pads (electrodes)
- Analysis capability
- Defibrillation capability
- Prompts to guide you
- Battery operation for portability

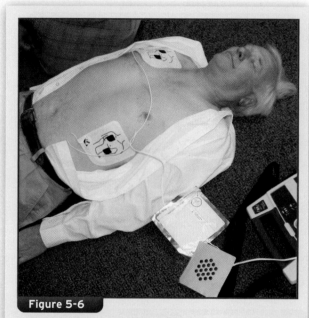

Figure 5-6

Two adhesive pads are placed on the victim's chest and connected by a cable to the AED.

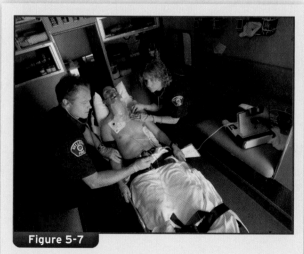

Figure 5-7

AEDs store data, including heart rhythms and shocks.

Using an AED

Once you have determined the need for the AED (victim unresponsive and not breathing), the basic operation of all AED models follows the sequence in **Skill Drill 5-1**.

Some AEDs power on by pressing an on/off button. Others power on when opening the AED case lid. Once the power is on, the AED will quickly go through some internal checks and will then begin to provide voice and screen prompts.

Expose the victim's chest. The skin must be fairly dry so that the pads will adhere and conduct electricity properly. If necessary, dry the skin with a towel. Because excessive chest hair may also interfere with adhesion and electrical conduction, you may need to quickly shave the area where the pads are to be placed.

Remove the backing from the pads and apply them firmly to the victim's bare chest according to the diagram on the pads. One pad is placed to the right of the breastbone, just below the collarbone and above the right nipple. The second pad is placed on the left side of the chest, left of the nipple and above the lower rib margin.

Make sure the cable is attached to the AED, and stand clear for analysis of the heart's electrical activity. No one should be in contact with the victim at this time, or later if a shock is indicated.

Verify that no one is in contact with the victim. The AED will advise of the need to shock and, depending on the device, will either advise the rescuer to push a button to administer the shock, or will deliver the shock automatically. Begin CPR immediately following the shock and follow the prompts that include reanalyzing the rhythm. If the shock worked, the victim will begin to regain signs of life. Continue providing care until EMS personnel arrive and take over.

Special Considerations

There are several special situations that you should be aware of when using an AED. These include the following:

- Water
- Children
- Medication patches
- Implanted devices

skill drill

5-1   Using an AED

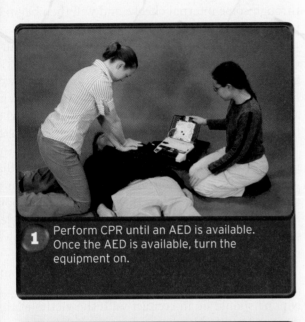

1 Perform CPR until an AED is available. Once the AED is available, turn the equipment on.

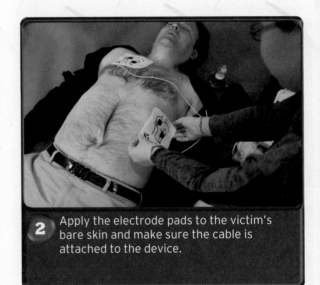

2 Apply the electrode pads to the victim's bare skin and make sure the cable is attached to the device.

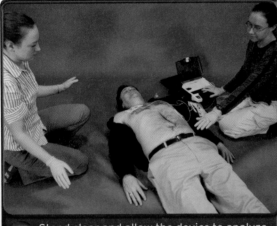
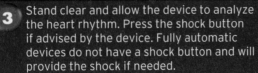

3 Stand clear and allow the device to analyze the heart rhythm. Press the shock button if advised by the device. Fully automatic devices do not have a shock button and will provide the shock if needed.

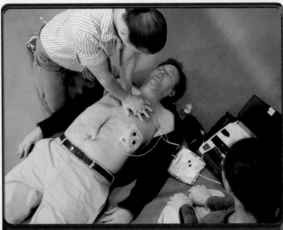

4 Perform CPR and follow the device prompts. Check the victim and repeat the analysis, shock, and CPR steps as needed.

Water

Because water conducts electricity, it may provide an energy pathway between the AED and the rescuer or bystanders. Remove the victim from free-standing water. Quickly dry the chest before applying the pads. The risk to the rescuers and bystanders is very low if the chest is dry and the pads are secured to the chest.

Children

Cardiac arrest in children is usually caused by an airway or breathing problem, rather than a primary heart problem as in adults. AEDs can deliver energy levels appropriate for children aged 1 year or older. If your AED has special pediatric pads and cable, use these for the child **Figure 5-8**. If the pediatric equipment is not available, use the adult equipment.

Medication Patches

Some people wear an adhesive patch containing medication (such as nitroglycerin, nicotine, or pain medication) that is absorbed through the skin. Because these patches may block the delivery of energy from the pads to the heart, they need to be removed and the skin wiped dry before attaching the AED pads **Figure 5-9**.

Implanted Devices

Implanted pacemakers and defibrillators are small devices placed underneath the skin of people with certain types of heart disease **Figure 5-10**. These devices can often be seen or felt when the chest is exposed. Avoid placing the pads directly over these devices whenever possible. If an implanted defibrillator is discharging, you may see the victim twitching periodically. Allow the implanted unit to stop before using your AED.

▶ AED Maintenance

Periodic inspection of your AED can ensure that the device has the necessary supplies and is in proper working condition **Figure 5-11**. AEDs conduct automatic internal checks and provide visual indications that the unit is ready and functioning properly. You do not need to turn the device on daily to check it as part of any inspection. Doing so will only wear down the battery.

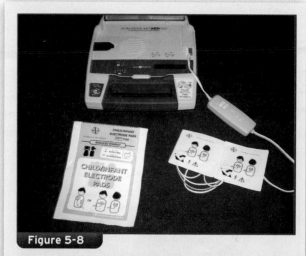

Figure 5-8

If your AED has pediatric pads, use them according to the manufacturer's instructions.

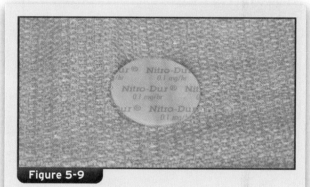

Figure 5-9

Remove any medication patches before applying AED pads.

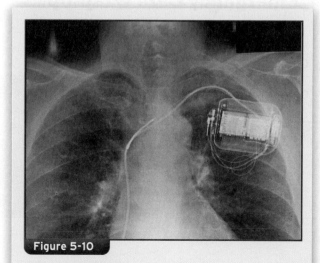

Figure 5-10

Implanted defibrillator.

AED supplies should include items such as the following:

- Two sets of electrode pads with expiration dates that are not expired
- Extra battery
- Razor
- Hand towel

Other items that should be considered are a breathing device (for example, a mask or shield) and medical exam gloves.

▶ AED Manufacturers

AED devices and related supplies are available from different manufacturers Figure 5-12 .

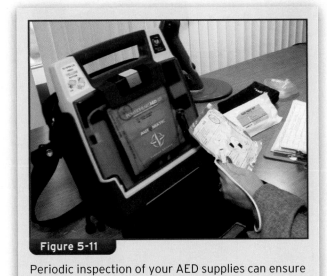

Figure 5-11

Periodic inspection of your AED supplies can ensure that all items are in working condition.

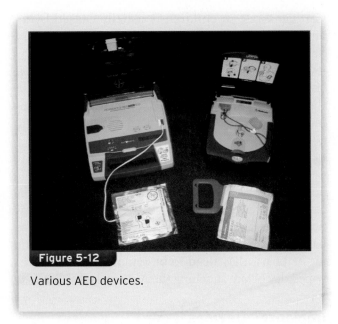

Figure 5-12

Various AED devices.

▶ Emergency Care Wrap-Up

Condition	What to Look For	What to Do
Cardiac arrest	• Unresponsiveness	1. Perform CPR until an AED is available. 2. Turn on the AED. 3. Apply the pads. 4. Analyze the heart rhythm. 5. Administer a shock if needed. 6. Perform CPR for five cycles (2 minutes). 7. Reanalyze and follow prompts.

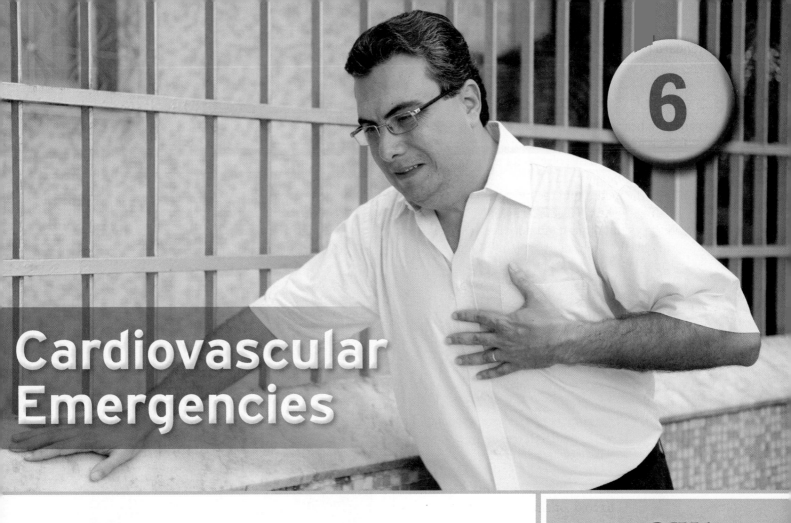

Cardiovascular Emergencies

6

▶ Heart Attack

A <u>heart attack</u> occurs when the heart muscle tissue dies because its blood supply is reduced or stopped. Usually a clot in a coronary artery (the vessel that carries blood to the heart muscle) blocks the blood supply. The heart may stop (known as cardiac arrest) if certain areas of the heart or too much heart muscle is damaged.

> **heart attack**
> Death of a part of the heart muscle.

Recognizing a Heart Attack

Prompt medical care at the onset of a heart attack is vital to survival and the quality of recovery. This is sometimes easier said than done because many victims deny they are experiencing something as serious as a heart attack. The signs of a heart attack include the following:

- Chest pressure, squeezing, or pain that lasts more than a few minutes or that goes away and comes back. Some victims have no chest pain.
- Pain spreading to the shoulders, neck, jaw, or arms
- Dizziness, sweating, nausea
- Shortness of breath

Many women do not have the classic signs of heart attack seen in men. Instead, they often have severe fatigue, upset stomach, and shortness of breath. Only about one third of women report of severe chest pain. While cardiovascular disease affects both sexes equally, when women have heart attacks they are more likely than men to die.

Meeting OSHA Recommendations

This chapter and the accompanying lesson cover the following *OSHA Best Practices Guide: Fundamentals of a Workplace First-Aid Program (2006)*:

4. Responding to Life-Threatening Emergencies
- Chest Pain
- Stroke

Care for a Heart Attack

To care for a heart attack victim:

1. Seek medical care by calling 9-1-1. Medications to dissolve a clot are available but must be given early.
2. Help the victim into the most comfortable resting position Figure 6-1 .
3. If the victim is alert and not allergic to aspirin, give four chewable aspirin (81 mg) or 1 regular aspirin (325 mg).
4. If the victim has prescribed medication for heart disease, such as nitroglycerin, help the victim use it.
5. Monitor breathing.

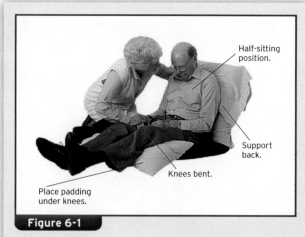

Figure 6-1

Half-sitting position.

Support back.

Knees bent.

Place padding under knees.

Help the victim into a relaxed position to ease strain on the heart.

▶ Angina

angina
Chest pain caused by a lack of blood to the heart muscle.

<u>Angina</u> is chest pain associated with heart disease that occurs when the heart muscle does not get enough blood. Angina is brought on by physical activity, exposure to cold, or emotional stress.

Recognizing Angina

The signs of angina are similar to those of a heart attack, but the pain seldom lasts longer than 10 minutes and almost always is relieved by nitroglycerin (a prescribed medication).

Care for Angina

To care for a victim with angina:

1. Have the victim rest.
2. If a victim has his or her own nitroglycerin, help the victim use it.
3. If the pain continues beyond 10 minutes, suspect a heart attack and call 9-1-1.

▶ Stroke

stroke
A blockage or rupture of arteries in the brain.

A <u>stroke</u>, also called a brain attack, occurs when part of the blood flow to the brain is suddenly cut off. This occurs when arteries in the brain rupture or become blocked Figure 6-2 .

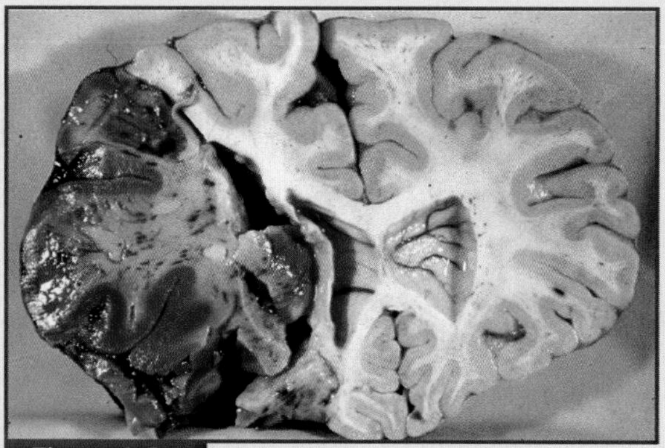

Figure 6-2

Severe brain hemorrhage causing a stroke.

Recognizing Stroke

The signs of a stroke include the following:

- Sudden weakness or numbness of the face, an arm, or a leg on one side of the body
- Blurred or decreased vision
- Problems speaking
- Dizziness or loss of balance
- Sudden, severe headache
- Sudden confusion

To assess for a possible stroke, you can use the mnemonic FAST Table 6-1 .

Table 6-1 Recognizing a Stroke

Face	Ask the person to smile. Does one side of the face droop?
Arms	Ask the person to extend both arms out. Does one arm drift downward?
Speech	Ask the person to repeat a simple sentence. Are the words slurred? Can the person repeat the sentence correctly?
Time	If the person shows any of these signs, time is important. Remember when the signs and symptoms first began. Do not lose any more time. Call 9-1-1 to get to a hospital promptly.

Care for Stroke

To care for a stroke victim:

1. Call 9-1-1.
2. Have the victim rest in a comfortable position. This is often on the back with the head and shoulders elevated.
3. If vomiting, roll the victim to his or her side (recovery position).

▶ Emergency Care Wrap-Up

Condition	What to Look For	What to Do
Heart attack	• Chest pressure, squeezing, or pain • Pain spreading to shoulders, neck, jaw, or arms • Dizziness, sweating, nausea • Shortness of breath	1. Help victim take his or her prescribed medication. 2. Call 9-1-1. 3. Help victim into a comfortable position. 4. If the victim is alert and not allergic to aspirin, give four chewable aspirin or one regular aspirin. 5. Assist with any prescribed heart medication. 6. Monitor breathing.
Angina	• Chest pain similar to a heart attack • Pain seldom lasts longer than 10 minutes	1. Have victim rest. 2. If victim has his or her own nitroglycerin, help the victim use it. 3. If pain continues beyond 10 minutes, suspect a heart attack and call 9-1-1.
Stroke	• Sudden weakness or numbness of the face, an arm, or a leg on one side of the body • Blurred or decreased vision • Problems speaking • Dizziness or loss of balance • Sudden, severe headache	1. Call 9-1-1. 2. Have the victim rest in a comfortable position. 3. If vomiting, roll the victim to his or her side.

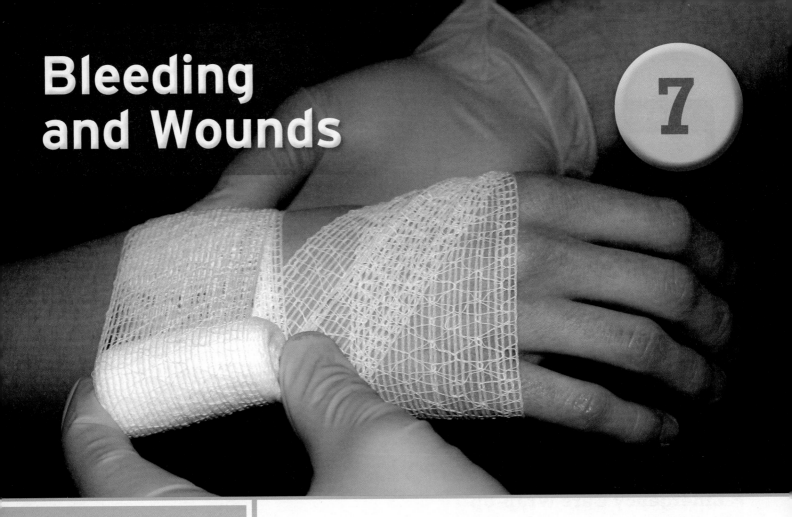

Bleeding and Wounds

7

Meeting OSHA Recommendations

This chapter and the accompanying lesson cover the following *OSHA Best Practices Guide: Fundamentals of a Workplace First-Aid Program (2006)*:

4. **Responding to Life-Threatening Emergencies**
   - Controlling bleeding with direct pressure.

5. **Responding to Non-Life-Threatening Emergencies**
   - Wounds
     - Assessment and first aid for wounds including abrasions, cuts, lacerations, punctures, avulsions, amputations, and crush injuries;
     - Principles of wound care, including infection precautions.
   - Musculoskeletal Injuries
     - Appropriate handling of amputated body parts.

▶ External Bleeding

> **hemorrhage**
> A large amount of bleeding in a short time.

External bleeding refers to when blood can be seen coming from an open wound. The term **hemorrhage** refers to a large amount of bleeding in a short time.

Recognizing External Bleeding

Injuries damage blood vessels and cause bleeding. The three types of bleeding relate to the type of blood vessel that is damaged: capillary, vein, or artery **Figure 7-1**.

> **capillary bleeding**
> Bleeding that oozes from a wound steadily but slowly.
>
> **venous bleeding**
> Bleeding from a vein; this type of bleeding tends to flow steadily.
>
> **arterial bleeding**
> Bleeding from an artery; this type of bleeding tends to spurt with each heartbeat.

- **Capillary bleeding** oozes slowly from a wound. It is the most common type of bleeding and easiest to control.
- **Venous bleeding** flows steadily. Because it is under less pressure, it does not spurt and is easier to control than arterial bleeding. However, large amounts of blood can be lost.
- **Arterial bleeding** spurts with each heartbeat. The pressure that causes the blood to spurt also makes this type of bleeding difficult to control. This is the most serious type of bleeding because a large amount of blood can be lost in a very short time.

There are several types of open wounds
Figure 7-2A–F:

- *Abrasion:* The top layer of skin is removed, with little blood loss. Other names for an abrasion are *scrape, road rash,* and *rug burn.*
- *Laceration:* Cut skin with jagged edges. This type of wound is usually caused by a forceful tearing away of skin tissue.
- *Incision:* A cut with smooth edges, such as a knife or paper cut.
- *Puncture:* Injury from a sharp, pointed object (such as a knife or bullet). The penetrating object can damage internal organs. The risk of infection is high. The object causing the injury may remain embedded (impaled) in the wound.

- *Avulsion:* A piece of skin and/or tissue torn loose and hanging from the body.
- *Amputation:* The cutting or tearing off of a body part.

Care for External Bleeding

Care for serious external bleeding involves controlling the bleeding and protecting the wound from further injury **Skill Drill 7-1**.

A minor (shallow) wound should be cleaned to help prevent infection. Wound cleaning usually restarts bleeding by disturbing the clot, but it should be done anyway. For severe bleeding, leave the pressure bandage in place until the victim can get medical care. To care for a shallow wound:

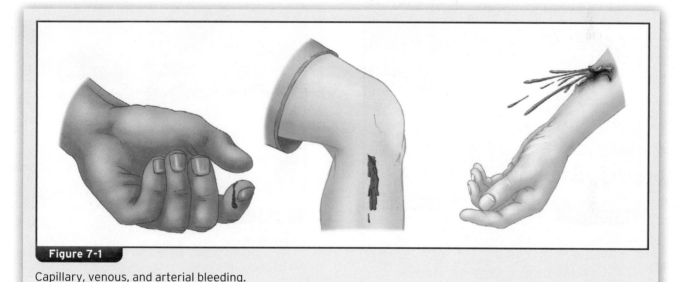

Figure 7-1

Capillary, venous, and arterial bleeding.

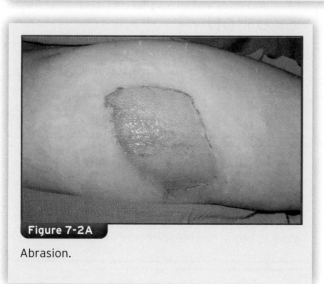

Figure 7-2A

Abrasion.

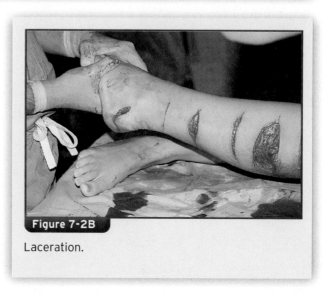

Figure 7-2B

Laceration.

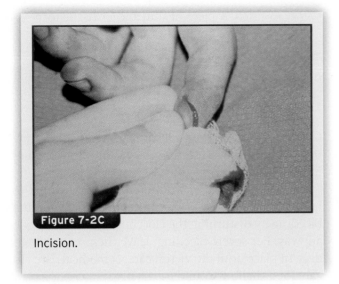

Figure 7-2C

Incision.

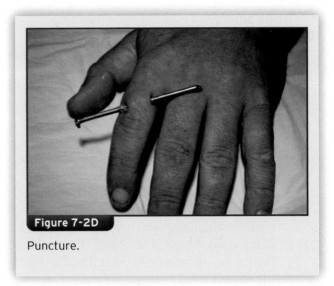

Figure 7-2D

Puncture.

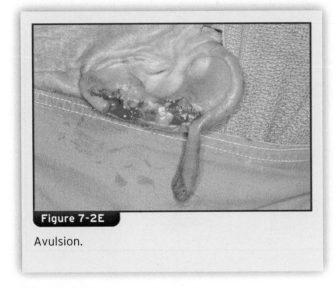

Figure 7-2E

Avulsion.

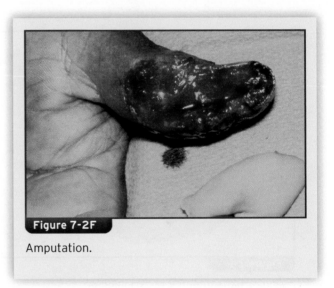

Figure 7-2F

Amputation.

1. If available, put on medical gloves.
2. Wash the wound with soap and water.
3. Flush the wound with running water under pressure.
4. Apply an antibiotic ointment.
5. Cover the area with a sterile and, if possible, nonstick dressing. Change the dressing and bandage periodically.
6. Seek medical care for a wound with a high risk for infection (such as an animal bite or a puncture).

CAUTION

Once the wound has been cared for, wash your hands with soap and water, even if you used medical exam gloves.

DO NOT use direct pressure on an eye injury, a wound with an embedded object, or a skull fracture.

CAUTION

DO NOT pull a scab loose to change the dressing. If a sticking dressing must be removed, soak it in warm water to help soften the scab and make removal easier.

skill drill

7-1   Care for Serious External Bleeding

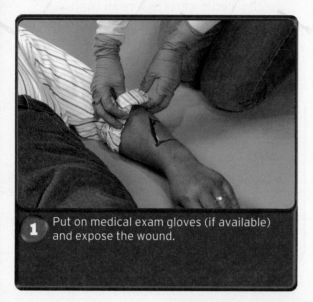

1 Put on medical exam gloves (if available) and expose the wound.

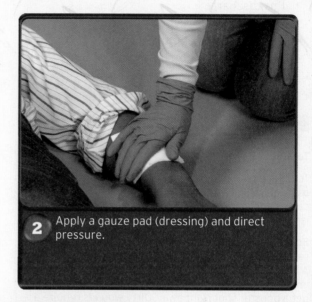

2 Apply a gauze pad (dressing) and direct pressure.

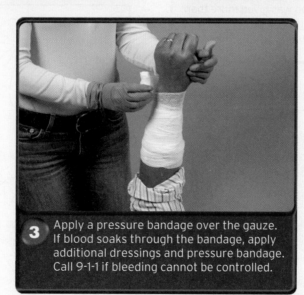

3 Apply a pressure bandage over the gauze. If blood soaks through the bandage, apply additional dressings and pressure bandage. Call 9-1-1 if bleeding cannot be controlled.

▶ Wound Infection

Any wound, large or small, can become infected **Figure 7-3**. Seek medical care for infected wounds.

The signs that a wound may be infected include the following:

- Swelling and redness around the wound
- A sensation of warmth
- Throbbing pain
- Pus discharge
- Fever
- Swelling of lymph nodes
- Red streaks leading from the wound toward the heart

FYI

Tetanus

Tetanus is caused by a bacterium that can produce a powerful toxin when it enters a wound. The toxin causes contractions of certain muscle groups, particularly in the jaw. There is no known cure for the toxin.

Because of this danger, everyone needs an initial series of vaccinations to defend against the toxin. A booster shot every 10 years is sufficient to maintain immunity, although anyone with an animal bite should get a booster shot right away. Dirty wounds require a booster shot if the immunization was given more than 5 years ago. Tetanus immunization shots must be given within 72 hours of the injury to be effective.

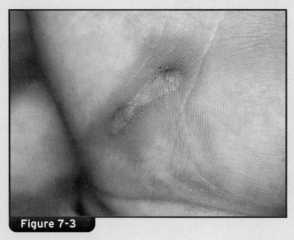

Figure 7-3
Infected wound.

▶ Amputations

The loss of a body part is a devastating injury that requires immediate medical care. To care for an amputation **Figure 7-4**:

1. Call 9-1-1.
2. Control bleeding.
3. Care for shock (see Chapter 8, *Shock*).
4. Recover the amputated part and wrap it in dry sterile gauze or a clean cloth.
5. Seal the wrapped amputated part in a plastic bag or other waterproof container.
6. Keep the part cool (for example, ice and water in a bowl), but do not freeze.

FYI

Cooling Amputated Parts

Amputated body parts that remain uncooled for more than 6 hours have little chance of survival; 18 hours is probably the maximum time allowable for a part that has been cooled properly. Muscles without blood lose viability within 4 to 6 hours.

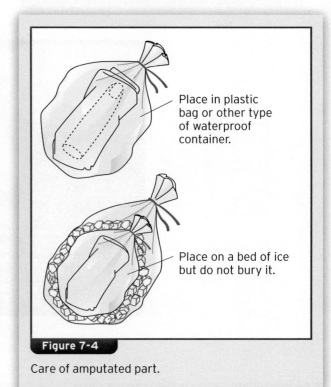

Place in plastic bag or other type of waterproof container.

Place on a bed of ice but do not bury it.

Figure 7-4
Care of amputated part.

▶ Impaled Objects

Objects such as glass, knives, and nails can be impaled (embedded) in the body **Figure 7-5**. To care for these wounds:

1. Leave the object in place.
2. Expose the area. Remove or cut away clothing surrounding the injury.
3. Stabilize the object with bulky dressings or clean cloths around the object.
4. Seek medical care.

▶ Wounds That Require Medical Care

There are some guidelines that can help you identify which wounds need emergency medical care.

- Wounds that will not stop bleeding after 5 minutes of applying direct pressure.
- Long or deep cuts that need sutures (stitches).
- Cuts over a joint.
- Cuts that may impair function of a body area such as an eyelid or lip.
- Cuts that remove all of the layers of the skin, such as those from slicing off the tip of a finger.
- Cuts from an animal or human bite.
- Cuts that have damaged underlying nerves, tendons, or joints.
- Cuts over a possible broken bone.
- Cuts caused by a crushing injury.
- Cuts with an object embedded in them.
- Cuts caused by a metal or glass object or a puncture wound.

Call 9-1-1 immediately if:

- Bleeding is not controlled with the application of pressure after 10–15 minutes.
- Signs of shock occur, such as dizziness and pale, cool skin.
- Breathing is difficult because of a cut to the neck or chest.
- A deep cut to the abdomen causes moderate to severe pain.
- The eyeball has been cut.
- A cut amputates or partially amputates an extremity.

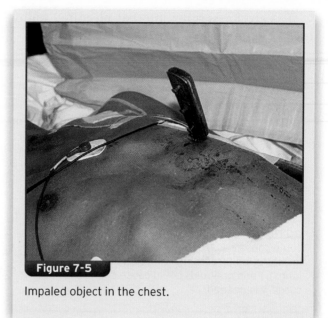

Figure 7-5

Impaled object in the chest.

▶ Internal Bleeding

A closed wound results when a blunt object does not break the skin, but tissue and blood vessels beneath the skin's surface are crushed, causing internal bleeding. In some cases it is easy to detect closed wounds from the bruising that often occurs. In other cases, a closed wound can be difficult to detect but can still be life threatening.

Recognizing Internal Bleeding

The signs of internal bleeding may appear quickly or take days to appear:

- Bruising
- Painful, tender area
- Vomiting or coughing up blood
- Stool that is black or contains bright red blood

Care for Internal Bleeding

For minor internal bleeding (such as a bruise on the leg from bumping into the corner of a table), follow these steps:

1. Apply ice or cold pack on the injured area for 20 minutes.
2. Compress the injured area by applying an elastic bandage for 2–3 hours.
3. Elevate an injured arm or leg, if it is not broken.
4. Repeat these steps.

To care for serious internal bleeding, follow these steps:

1. Call 9-1-1.
2. Care for shock by placing the victim on his or her back and covering the victim to maintain warmth.
3. If vomiting occurs, roll the victim onto his or her side to keep the airway clear.
4. Monitor breathing.

CAUTION

DO NOT give a victim anything to eat or drink. It could cause nausea and vomiting, which could result in aspiration (breathing in foreign material into the lungs). Food or liquids could cause complications if surgery is needed.

▶ Dressings and Bandages

dressing
A sterile gauze pad or clean cloth covering placed over an open wound.

First aid kits include dressings and bandages to be used when controlling bleeding and caring for wounds. A **dressing** is a covering that is placed directly over a wound to help absorb blood, prevent infection, and protect the wound from further injury. Dressings come in different shapes, sizes, and types. Dressings can be gauze pads (for example, 2″ or 4″ square or larger) used to cover larger wounds, or adhesive strips such as Band-Aids, which are dressings combined with a bandage for small cuts or scrapes **Figure 7-6**.

bandage
Used to cover a dressing to keep it in place on the wound and to apply pressure to help control bleeding.

A **bandage**, such as a roll of gauze, is often used to cover a dressing to keep it in place on the wound and to apply pressure to help control the bleeding. Like dressings, bandages also come in different shapes, sizes, and material **Figure 7-7**. Elastic bandages can be used to provide support and stability for an extremity or joint and to reduce swelling.

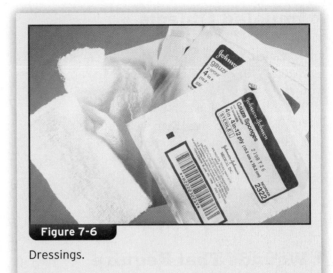
Figure 7-6
Dressings.

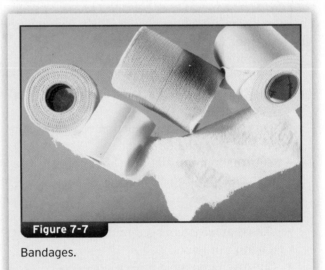
Figure 7-7
Bandages.

FYI

Sutures (Stitches)

If sutures are needed, they should be placed by a physician, usually within 6 to 8 hours of the injury. Suturing wounds allows faster healing, reduces infection, and lessens scarring.

Some wounds do not usually require sutures:

• Wounds in which the skin's cut edges tend to fall together

• Shallow cuts less than 1″ long

Rather than close a gaping wound with butterfly bandages, cover the wound with sterile gauze. Closing the wound might trap bacteria inside, resulting in an infection. In most cases, a physician can be reached in time for sutures to be placed. Gaping wounds should be evaluated by a medical professional.

▶ Emergency Care Wrap-Up

Condition	What to Look For	What to Do
Serious external bleeding	• Large amount of blood coming from an open wound	1. Put on medical exam gloves (if available) and expose the wound. 2. Apply a gauze pad (dressing) and direct pressure. 3. Apply a pressure bandage over the gauze. 4. If blood soaks through the bandage, apply additional dressings and pressure bandage. 5. Call 9-1-1 if bleeding cannot be controlled.

Internal bleeding	• Bruising
	• Painful, tender area
	• Vomiting or coughing up blood
	• Stool that is black or contains bright red blood
		Minor internal bleeding:
		1. Follow these procedures:
		  R = Rest
		  I = Ice or cold pack
		  C = Compress the area with elastic bandage
		  E = Elevate if the extremity is injured
		
		Serious internal bleeding:
		1. Call 9-1-1.
		2. Care for shock.
		3. If vomiting occurs, roll the victim onto side.

Minor wound	• Small amount of bleeding	1. Wash with soap and water. 2. Flush with running water under pressure. 3. Apply antibiotic ointment. 4. Cover with sterile or clean dressing. 5. For wounds with a high risk for infection, seek medical care for cleaning, possible tetanus booster, and closing.
Wound infection	• Swelling and redness around the wound • Sensation of warmth • Throbbing pain • Pus discharge • Fever • Swelling of lymph nodes • Red streaks leading from the wound toward the heart	1. Seek medical care.
Amputation	• Loss of a body part	1. Call 9-1-1. 2. Control bleeding. 3. Care for shock. 4. Recover amputated part(s) and wrap in sterile or clean dressing. 5. Seal wrapped part(s) in a plastic bag or waterproof container. 6. Keep part(s) cool, but not frozen.
Impaled object	• Object remains in wound	1. Do not remove object. 2. Stabilize the object with bulky dressings or clean cloths.

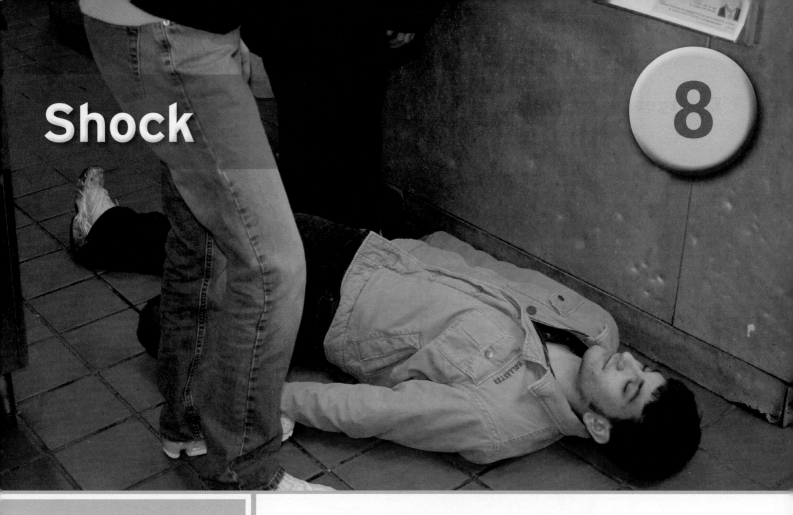

Shock

8

Meeting ⊙SHA Recommendations

This chapter and the accompanying lesson cover the following *OSHA Best Practices Guide: Fundamentals of a Workplace First-Aid Program (2006)*:

4. Responding to Life-Threatening Emergencies
- Recognizing the signs and symptoms of shock and providing first aid for shock due to illness or injury.

▶ Shock

> **shock**
> Inadequate tissue oxygenation resulting from serious injury or illness.

<u>Shock</u> occurs when the body's tissues do not receive enough oxygenated blood. Do not confuse this with an electric shock or "being shocked," as in being scared or surprised. To understand shock, think of the circulatory system as having three components: a working pump (the heart), a network of pipes (the blood vessels), and an adequate amount of fluid (the blood) pumped through the pipes. Damage to any of the components can deprive tissues of oxygen-rich blood and produce the condition known as shock.

Recognizing Shock

The signs of shock include the following:
- Altered mental status:
  - Agitation
  - Anxiety
  - Restlessness
  - Confusion
- Pale or bluish, cold, and clammy skin, lips, and nail beds
- Nausea and vomiting
- Rapid breathing
- Unresponsiveness (when shock is severe)

Care for Shock

To care for shock:
1. Place the victim on his or her back **Figure 8-1** .
2. Keep the victim warm.
3. Call 9-1-1.

FYI

If the victim is vomiting, has heavy secretions, or if you must leave an unresponsive victim to call 9-1-1, roll the victim onto his or her side to allow the vomit or secretions to drain from the victim's mouth and to keep the airway clear.

▶ Anaphylactic Reaction

anaphylaxis
A life-threatening allergic reaction.

A life-threatening breathing emergency can result from a severe allergic reaction called **anaphylaxis**. This reaction happens when a substance to which the victim is very sensitive enters the body. It can be deadly within minutes if untreated. Many of the deaths are caused by the inability to breathe because swollen airway passages block air to the lungs. The most common causes of anaphylaxis include the following:
- Medications (for example, penicillin and related drugs, aspirin, sulfa drugs)
- Food (for example, nuts, especially peanuts; eggs; shellfish)
- Insect stings (for example, honeybee, yellow jacket, wasp, hornet, fire ant)
- Plants (for example, inhaled pollen)

Recognizing Anaphylaxis

The most common signs of anaphylaxis include the following:
- Breathing difficulty—shortness of breath and wheezing
- Skin reaction—itching or burning skin, especially over the face and upper part of the chest, with rash or hives
- Swelling of the tongue, mouth, or throat

Other signs of anaphylaxis can include:
- Sneezing, coughing
- Tightness in the chest
- Blueness around lips and mouth
- Dizziness
- Nausea and vomiting

Care for Anaphylaxis

To care for anaphylaxis:
1. Call 9-1-1.
2. Determine if the victim has medication for allergic reactions. If the victim has a prescribed **epinephrine auto-injector** **Figure 8-2** , help the victim use it. If you are assisting with or using an auto-injector, follow the steps in **Skill Drill 8-1** .

   epinephrine auto-injector
   Prescribed device used to administer an emergency dose of epinephrine to a victim experiencing anaphylaxis.

3. Keep a responsive victim sitting up to help breathing. Place an unresponsive victim on his or her back (or side if vomiting occurs).

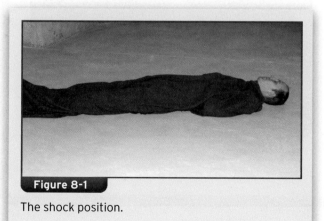

Figure 8-1
The shock position.

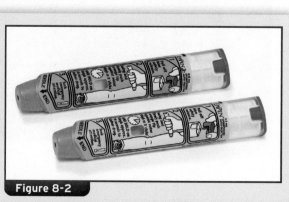

Figure 8-2
Prescribed epinephrine auto-injectors.

FYI

Epinephrine: A Lifesaver

Epinephrine constricts blood vessels and elevates blood pressure, dilates passages in the lungs to make breathing easier, and makes the heart beat stronger. These all help the anaphylaxis victim.

People who have severe allergic reactions may have a physician-prescribed epinephrine auto-injector, and may also need assistance with its use in an emergency. Two types of injectors are available:

- EpiPen (can only give 1 dose)
- Twinject (can give 2 doses)

Each device is available in both adult and child dosages.

Epinephrine should be used only when the victim is showing signs of a severe allergic reaction, especially difficulty breathing.

skill drill

8-1   Using an Epinephrine Auto-Injector

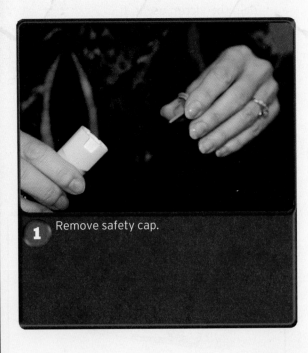

1 Remove safety cap.

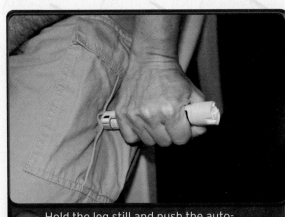

2 Hold the leg still and push the auto-injector against the thigh. Hold in place for 10 seconds. It is best to expose the skin of the thigh, but do not delay injection if it is not possible to quickly expose the skin. Reinsert used auto-injector, needle first, into the carrying tube.

▶ Emergency Care Wrap-Up

Condition	What to Look For	What to Do
Shock	• Altered mental status (anxiety, restlessness; confusion) • Pale, cold, and clammy skin, lips, and nail beds • Nausea and vomiting • Rapid breathing	1. Place the victim on his or her back. 2. Keep the victim warm. 3. Call 9-1-1.
Anaphylaxis	• Breathing difficulty • Skin reaction • Swelling of the tongue, mouth, or throat • Sneezing, coughing • Tightness in the chest • Blueness around lips and mouth • Dizziness • Nausea and vomiting	1. Call 9-1-1. 2. Determine if victim has a prescribed epinephrine auto-injector and help the victim use it. 3. Keep a responsive victim sitting up to help breathing. Place an unresponsive victim on his or her back (or side if vomiting ocurs).

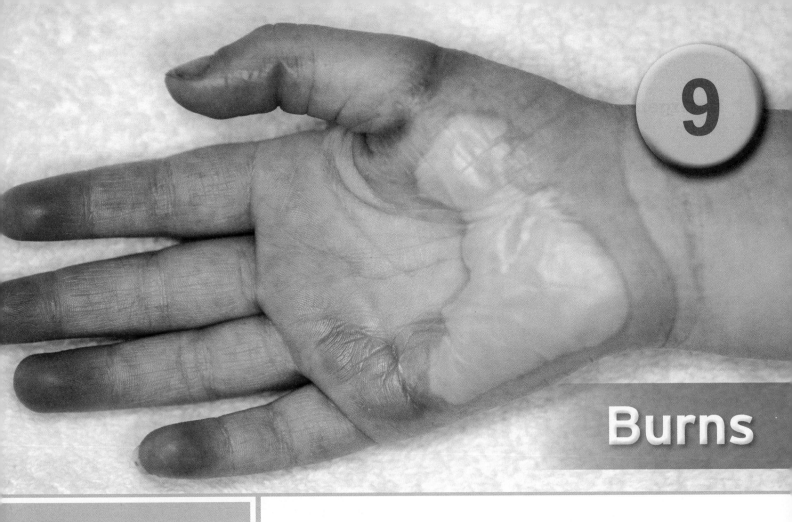

Burns

9

Meeting OSHA Recommendations

This chapter and the accompanying lesson cover the following *OSHA Best Practices Guide: Fundamentals of a Workplace First-Aid Program (2006):*

5. Responding to Non-Life-Threatening Emergencies

- Burns
  - Assessing the severity of a burn;
  - Recognizing whether a burn is thermal, electrical, or chemical and the appropriate first aid;
  - Reviewing corrosive chemicals at a specific worksite, along with appropriate first aid.

▶ Types of Burns

Burn injuries can be classified as thermal (heat), chemical, or electrical.

- *Thermal (heat) burns.* Thermal burns can be caused by flames, contact with hot objects, flammable vapor that ignites and causes a flash or an explosion, steam, or hot liquid.
- *Chemical burns.* Chemical agents can cause tissue damage and death if they come in contact with the skin. Three types of chemicals—acids, alkalis, and organic compounds—are responsible for most chemical burns.
- *Electrical burns.* The severity of injury from contact with electric current depends on the type of current (direct or alternating), the voltage, the area of the body exposed, and the duration of contact.

▶ Depth of Burns

Determine the depth (degree) of the burn. Historically, burns have been described as first-degree, second-degree, and third-degree injuries. Medical care professionals use the terms *superficial, partial thickness,* and *full thickness* because they are more descriptive of the extent of tissue damage.

- **First-degree (superficial) burns** affect the skin's outer layer (epidermis) **Figure 9-1**. Characteristics include redness, mild swelling, tenderness, and pain. Sunburn is a common example of a first-degree burn. Healing occurs without scarring, usually within a week.

- **Second-degree (partial-thickness) burns** extend through the skin's entire outer layer and into the inner layer **Figure 9-2**. Blisters, swelling, weeping of fluids, and pain identify these burns. Intact blisters provide a sterile, waterproof covering. Once a blister breaks, a weeping wound results, and the risk of infection increases. Large second-degree burns require medical care.

- **Third-degree (full-thickness) burns** are severe burns that penetrate all the skin layers and the underlying fat and muscle **Figure 9-3**. The skin looks leathery, waxy, or pearly gray, and sometimes charred. A third-degree burn requires medical care.

If a burn wraps all the way around a body part, such as a finger, toe, arm, or torso, this is a circumferential burn. A circumferential burn requires medical care.

▶ Extent of Burns

Part of determining the severity of a burn requires you to estimate how much body surface area the burn covers. You can use the Rule of the Hand to estimate the size of a burn. The victim's entire hand represents about 1% of his or her total Body Surface Area (BSA) **Figure 9-4**.

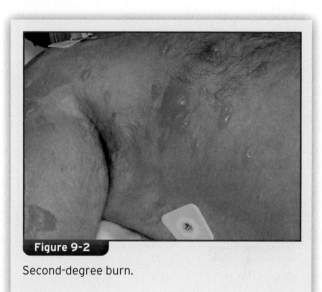

Figure 9-2

Second-degree burn.

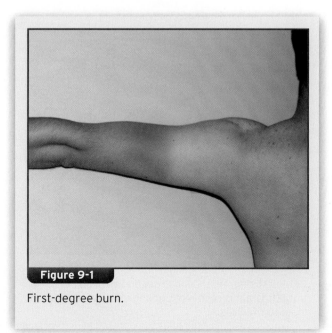

Figure 9-1

First-degree burn.

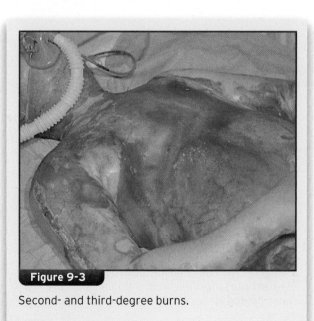

Figure 9-3

Second- and third-degree burns.

Determine which parts of the body are burned. Burns on the face, hands, feet, and genitals are more severe than on other body parts.

Determine whether other injuries or preexisting medical problems are present or if the victim is elderly or very young. A medical problem or belonging to one of these age groups increases a burn's severity.

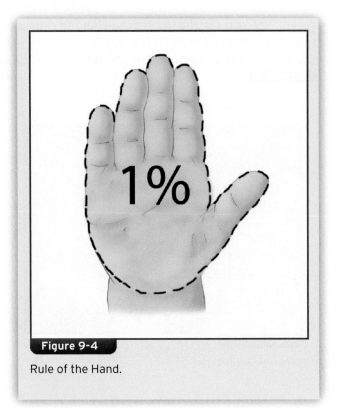

Figure 9-4

Rule of the Hand.

FYI

Respiratory Injuries

Inhaling air at a temperature above 300°F can cause death in minutes. The air temperature near the ceiling of a burning room may reach temperatures of 1,000°F or higher.

Death can occur when the mucous membranes lining the respiratory system secrete fluids that fill the lungs. Victims of heat inhalation can actually drown in their own secretions.

Damage from inhaling the super-heated air may cause swelling of the respiratory tract. As with burns of the skin, swelling does not occur immediately after the injury: The risk of airway obstruction is greatest 12 to 24 hours after the burn. All victims exposed to super-heated air require medical care.

▶ Care for Thermal Burns

Burn care aims to reduce pain, protect against infection, and determine the need for medical care. Most burns are minor and can be managed without medical care. If clothing is burning, have the victim roll on the ground using the "stop, drop, and roll" method. Smother the flames with a blanket or douse the victim with water.

Care for First-Degree Burns

1. Cool the burn with cool water until the part is pain free (this often takes 10 minutes) **Figure 9-5**.
2. After the burn cools, apply an aloe vera gel or skin moisturizer to keep the skin moistened and to reduce itching and peeling.
3. Give an over-the-counter pain medication such as ibuprofen.

Care for Small Second-Degree Burns (<10% BSA)

1. Cool the burn with cool water until the part is pain free (often takes 10 minutes).
2. After the burn has been cooled, apply anti-biotic ointment. Do not apply lotions or aloe vera.
3. Cover the burn loosely with a dry, nonstick, sterile or clean dressing. Do not break any blisters.

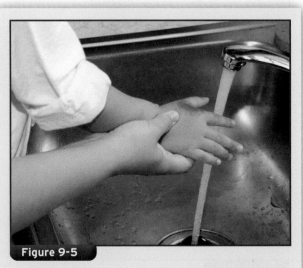

Figure 9-5

Cool first-degree and small second-degree burns until the pain is relieved. Cooling usually takes at least 10 minutes.

4. Give an over-the-counter pain medication such as ibuprofen.
5. Seek medical care.

Care for Large Second-Degree (≥20% BSA) and All Third-Degree Burns

1. Remove clothing and jewelry that are not stuck to the burned area.
2. Cover the burn loosely with a dry, nonstick, sterile or clean dressing.
3. Care for shock.
4. Call 9-1-1.

▶ Chemical Burns

A chemical burn results when a caustic or corrosive substance touches the skin **Figure 9-6** . Examples of such substances include acids, alkalis, and organic compounds. Because chemicals continue to burn as long as they are in contact with the skin, they should be removed from the skin as rapidly as possible.

First aid is the same for most chemical burns, except for a few specific ones for which a chemical neutralizer has to be used. Alkalis such as drain cleaners cause more serious burns than acids such as battery acid because they penetrate deeper and remain active longer. Organic compounds such as petroleum products are also capable of burning.

CAUTION

DO NOT apply water under high pressure—it will drive the chemical deeper into the tissue. Material Safety Data Sheets (MSDSs) provide information for handling particular substances and what to do if an incident occurs.

CAUTION

Put on medical exam gloves before helping a victim with chemical burns to protect your skin.

Care for Chemical Burns

1. Immediately flush the area with a large quantity of water for 20 minutes **Figure 9-7** . If the chemical is a dry powder, brush the powder from the skin before flushing with water **Figure 9-8** .
2. Remove the victim's contaminated clothing and jewelry while flushing with water.
3. Cover the affected area with a dry, sterile or clean dressing.
4. Seek medical care.

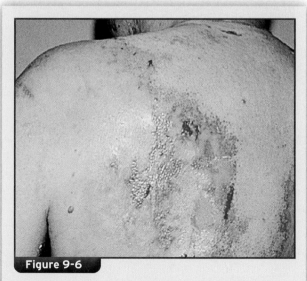

Figure 9-6

Chemical burn from sulfuric acid.

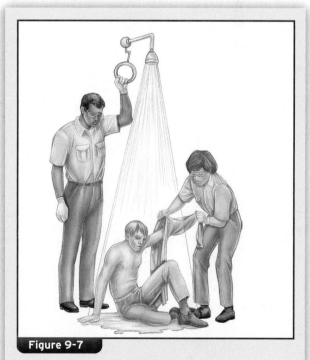

Figure 9-7

Flush a chemical burn with large amounts of running water.

▶ Electrical Burns

There are three types of electrical injuries: thermal burn (flame), arc burn (flash), and true electrical injury (contact). A thermal burn results when clothing or objects in contact with the skin are ignited by an electric current. These injuries are caused by the flames produced by the electric current, not by the passage of the electric current or arc.

An arc burn occurs when electricity jumps, or arcs, from one spot to another. Although the duration of the flash may be brief, it usually causes extensive superficial injuries.

A true electrical injury happens when an electric current passes directly through the body, which can disrupt the normal heart rhythm and cause cardiac arrest, other internal injuries, and burns. Usually, the electricity exits where the body touches a surface or comes in contact with a ground (for example, a metal object). This type of injury is often characterized by an entrance and exit wound Figure 9-9 .

Care for Electrical Burns

1. Make sure the area is safe. Unplug, disconnect, or turn off the power. If that is impossible, call 9-1-1.
2. Check responsiveness and breathing.
3. Provide CPR if necessary.
4. Care for shock.
5. Call 9-1-1.

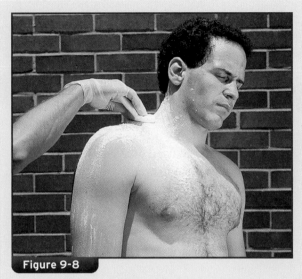

Figure 9-8

Brush dry chemicals off.

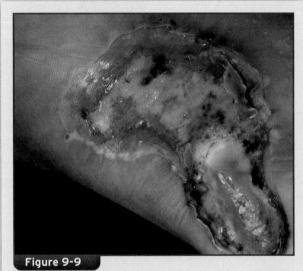

Figure 9-9

Electrical burn exit wound.

▶ Emergency Care Wrap-Up

Condition	What to Look For	What to Do
First-degree burn	• Redness • Mild swelling • Pain	1. Cool the burn with cool water. 2. Apply aloe vera gel or a skin moisturizer.
Small second-degree burn (<10% body surface area)	• Blisters • Swelling • Pain • Weeping of fluid	1. Cool the burn with cool water. 2. Apply antibiotic ointment. 3. Cover loosely with a dry, nonstick, sterile dressing. 4. If available, give an over-the-counter pain medication. 5. Seek medical care.
Large second-degree (≥10% body surface area) and third-degree burns	• Dry, leathery skin • Gray or charred skin	1. Cover burn loosely with a dry, nonstick, sterile or clean dressing. 2. Care for shock. 3. Call 9-1-1.
Chemical burns	• Stinging pain	1. Flush with a large amount of water for 20 minutes. 2. Remove victim's contaminated clothing and jewelry while flushing. 3. Seek medical care.
Electrical burns	• Possible third-degree burn with entrance and exit wounds	1. Unplug, disconnect, or turn off the electricity. 2. Check responsiveness and breathing. 3. Provide CPR if necessary. 4. Care for shock. 5. Call 9-1-1.

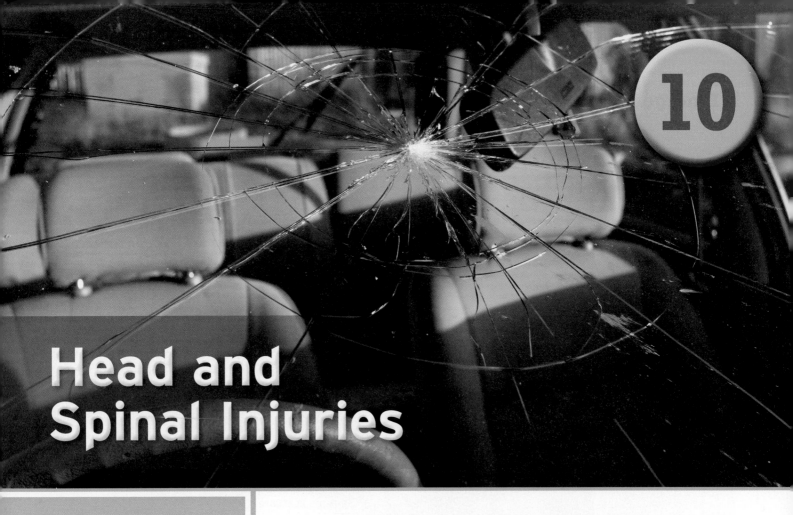

Head and Spinal Injuries

Meeting ⊙SHA Recommendations

This chapter and the accompanying lesson cover the following *OSHA Best Practices Guide: Fundamentals of a Workplace First-Aid Program (2006)*:

5. Responding to Non-Life-Threatening Emergencies
- Musculoskeletal Injuries
  - Head, neck, back and spinal injuries.
- Eye Injuries
  - First aid for eye injuries;
  - First aid for chemical burns.
- Mouth and Teeth Injuries
  - Oral injuries; lip and tongue injuries; broken and missing teeth;
  - The importance of preventing aspiration of blood and/or teeth.

Head Injuries

Any head injury is potentially serious. If not properly treated, injuries that seem minor could become life threatening. Head injuries include scalp wounds, skull fractures, and brain injuries. Spinal injuries (that is, neck and back injuries) can also be present in head-injured victims.

▶ Scalp Wounds

The scalp has many blood vessels, so any cut can cause heavy bleeding. A bleeding scalp wound does not affect the blood supply to the brain.

Care for Scalp Wounds

To care for a scalp wound:
1. Apply a sterile or clean dressing and direct pressure to control bleeding **Figure 10-1**.
2. Keep the victim's head and shoulders slightly elevated to help control bleeding if no spinal injury is suspected.
3. Seek medical care.

52

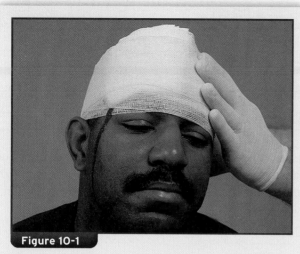

Figure 10-1

Apply direct pressure and a bandage to control bleeding.

FYI

There is no need to keep a concussion victim awake. This was previously recommended to observe a person for any changes after a concussion. The concern was that the victim may go into a coma; however, this is no longer believed to be true.

Once a person has had a concussion, he or she is as much as four times more likely to sustain a second one. After a concussion, it takes less of a blow to cause another concussion and requires more time to recover.

▶ Skull Fracture

skull fracture
A break of part of the skull (head bones).

Significant force applied to the head may cause a **skull fracture**. This occurs when part of the skull (the bones forming the head) is broken.

Recognizing Skull Fracture

Signs of skull fracture include the following:
- Pain at the point of injury
- A break in or deformity of the skull
- Loss of responsiveness
- Drainage of clear or bloody fluid from the ears or nose
- Heavy scalp bleeding (A scalp wound may expose the skull or brain tissue.)
- Penetrating wound, such as from a bullet or an impaled object

Care for Skull Fracture

To care for a skull fracture:
1. Check responsiveness and breathing and provide any necessary care.
2. Control any bleeding by applying a sterile or clean dressing and applying pressure around the edges of the wound, not directly on it Figure 10-2.
3. Stabilize the head and neck to prevent movement.
4. Call 9-1-1.

▶ Brain Injuries

The brain can be shaken by a blow to the head. A temporary disturbance of brain activity known as a **concussion** can result. Most concussions are mild, and people recover fully, but this process takes time. Concussions do not involve bleeding under the skull or swelling of brain tissue.

concussion
A temporary disturbance of brain activity caused by a blow to the head.

Recognizing Brain Injury

Signs of brain injury include the following:
- Befuddled facial expression (vacant stare)
- Slow to answer questions or follow directions
- Unaware of where they are or day of week (amnesia)
- Slurred speech
- Stumbling, inability to walk
- Loss of responsiveness
- Complaints of headache, dizziness, and nausea within minutes or hours of injury
- Making repetitive statements or asking the same questions over and over again

Care for Brain Injuries

To care for a brain injury:
1. Check responsiveness and breathing and provide any necessary care.
2. Stabilize the head and neck to prevent movement.
3. Control any scalp bleeding with a sterile or clean dressing and direct pressure. If you suspect a skull fracture, apply pressure around the wound edges, not directly on the wound.

4. If the victim vomits, roll the victim onto his or her side to keep the airway clear, moving the head, neck, and body as one unit.
5. Call 9-1-1.

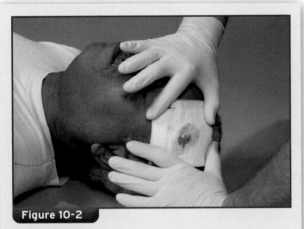

Figure 10-2

Apply pressure around the edges of the wound to control bleeding from a suspected skull fracture.

FYI

Head Injury Follow-up

Seek medical care if any of the following signs appear within 48 hours of a head injury. These symptoms can be caused by excessive pressure on or in the brain.

- **Headache:** Severe headache, or one that lasts more than 1 or 2 days or gets worse
- **Nausea, vomiting:** Nausea that does not go away, or vomiting more than once
- **Drowsiness and confusion**
- **Vision and eye problems:** Double vision, eyes that do not move together, one pupil that appears larger than the other, or dilated pupils (larger than normal)
- **Mobility:** Weakness, numbness in arms or legs, or trouble walking
- **Speech:** Slurred speech or inability to talk
- **Seizures (convulsions)**

CAUTION

DO NOT stop the flow of fluid from the ears or nose. Blocking the flow of either could increase pressure inside the skull.

DO NOT elevate the legs—that might increase pressure on the brain.

DO NOT clean an open skull injury—infection of the brain may result.

Eye Injuries

An eye injury can produce severe lifelong complications, including blindness if not treated promptly. When in doubt about an injury's severity, seek medical care.

▶ Foreign Objects in Eye

Many different types of objects can enter the eye and cause significant damage. Even a small foreign object, such as a grain of sand, can produce severe irritation.

Care for Loose Foreign Objects in the Eye

Try one or more of the following techniques to remove the object **Figure 10-3** :

1. Pull the upper lid over the lower lid, so that the lower lashes can brush the object off the inside of the upper lid.
2. Hold the eyelid open, and gently rinse with warm water.
3. Examine the lower lid by pulling it down gently. If you can see the object, remove it with moistened sterile gauze, clean cloth, or a moistened cotton swab.
4. Examine the underside of the upper lid by grasping the lashes of the upper lid and rolling the lid upward over a cotton swab. If you can see the object, remove it with moistened sterile gauze or a clean cloth.

CAUTION

DO NOT allow the victim to rub the eye.

DO NOT try to remove an embedded foreign object.

DO NOT use dry cotton (cotton balls or cotton-tipped swabs) or instruments such as tweezers to remove an object from an eye.

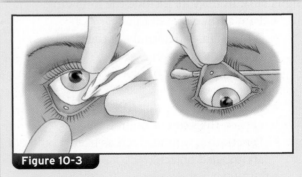

Figure 10-3

Locate and remove a foreign object from the eye.

▶ Penetrating Eye Injuries

Penetrating eye injuries result when a sharp object penetrates the eyeball and then is withdrawn or when an object remains embedded in the eye.

Care for Penetrating Eye Injuries

To care for a penetrating eye injury:
1. Stabilize long embedded objects with bulky dressings or clean cloths held in place Figure 10-4.
2. Ask the victim to close the uninjured eye.
3. Call 9-1-1.

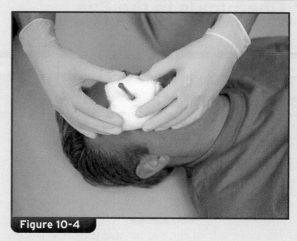

Figure 10-4

Protecting a penetrating object against movement with a bulky dressing.

▶ Blows to the Eye

Blows to the eye range from an ordinary black eye to severe damage that threatens eyesight Figure 10-5.

Care for Blows to the Eye

To care for a blow to the eye:
1. Apply an ice or cold pack for about 15 minutes to reduce pain and swelling. Do not apply it directly on the eyeball or apply any pressure on the eye.
2. Seek medical care if there is pain, double vision, reduced vision, or discoloration.

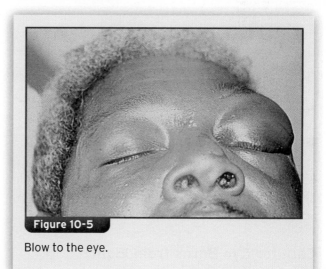

Figure 10-5

Blow to the eye.

▶ Eye Avulsion

eye avulsion
Forcible separation of the eyeball from its socket.

An **eye avulsion** occurs from a blow to the eye that knocks the eyeball from its socket.

Care for Eye Avulsion

To care for an eye avulsion:
1. Cover the injured eye loosely with a sterile or clean moistened dressing. Do not try to push the eyeball back into the socket.
2. Protect the injured eye with a paper cup, held in place by tape.
3. Have the victim keep the uninjured eye closed.
4. Call 9-1-1.

▶ Cuts of the Eye or Lid

Cuts of the eye or lid require very careful repair to restore appearance and function Figure 10-6.

Care for Cuts of the Eye or Lid

To care for a cut of the eye or lid:
1. If the eyeball is cut, do not apply pressure on it. If only the eyelid is cut, apply a sterile or clean dressing with gentle pressure.
2. Have the victim keep the uninjured eye closed.
3. Call 9-1-1.

▶ Chemicals in the Eye

Chemical burns of the eye, usually caused by an acid or alkaline solution, need immediate care because damage can occur in as little as 1 minute. They may cause loss of vision.

Care for Chemicals in the Eye

To care for a chemical in the eye:
1. Hold the eye wide open and flush with warm water for at least 20 minutes, continuously and gently **Figure 10-7**. Irrigate from the nose side of the eye toward the outside to avoid flushing material into the other eye.
2. Loosely bandage the eyes with wet dressings.
3. Call 9-1-1.

CAUTION

DO NOT try to neutralize the chemical. Water usually is readily available and is better for eye irrigation.

▶ Eye Burns from Light

Burns can result from looking at a source of ultraviolet light, such as a welder's arc or the glare off bright snow. Severe pain occurs several hours after exposure.

Care for Eye Burns from Light

To care for an eye burn from light:
1. Cover both eyes with wet dressings and cold packs. Tell the victim not to rub the eyes.
2. Seek medical care.

Nose Injuries

The nose often gets hit during sports activities, physical assaults, and motor vehicle crashes.

▶ Nosebleeds

Rupture of tiny blood vessels inside the nostrils by a blow to the nose, sneezing, or picking or blowing the nose causes most nosebleeds.

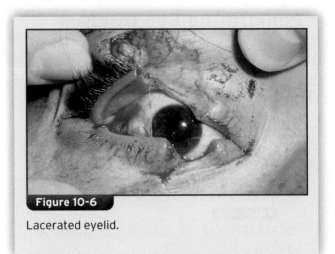

Figure 10-6

Lacerated eyelid.

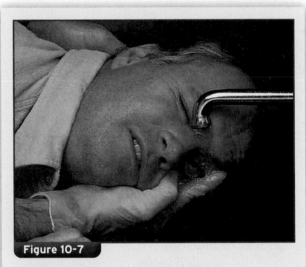

Figure 10-7

Flushing eye to treat a chemical burn.

There are two types of nosebleeds:
- **Anterior nosebleeds** (*front of nose*) are the most common type of nosebleed (90%) and are normally easily cared for.
- A **posterior nosebleed** (*back of nose*) involves massive bleeding backward into the mouth or down the back of the throat. A posterior nosebleed is serious and requires medical care.

anterior nosebleed
Bleeding from the front of the nose.

posterior nosebleed
Bleeding from the back of the nose into the mouth or down the back of the throat.

Care for Nosebleeds

To care for a nosebleed:
1. Place the victim in a seated position with the victim's head tilted slightly forward.
2. Pinch (or have the victim pinch) the soft parts of the nose between the thumb and two fingers with steady pressure for at least 5 to 10 minutes **Figure 10-8**.
3. Seek medical care if bleeding cannot be controlled or you suspect a broken nose.

▶ Broken Nose

A blow to the nose can break the nose.

Recognizing a Broken Nose

The signs of a broken nose include the following:
- Pain, swelling, or deformity
- Bleeding and breathing difficulty through the nostrils
- Black eyes appearing 1 to 2 days after the injury

Care for a Broken Nose

To care for a broken nose:
1. If bleeding, provide care as for a nosebleed.
2. Apply an ice or cold pack to the nose. Do not try to straighten a crooked nose.
3. Seek medical care.

Mouth Injuries

Mouth injuries can involve damage to the lips, tongue, and teeth. These injuries can cause considerable pain and anxiety.

▶ Bitten Lip or Tongue

Care for Bitten Lip or Tongue

To care for a bitten lip or tongue:
1. Apply direct pressure.
2. Apply an ice or cold pack.
3. If the bleeding does not stop, seek medical care.

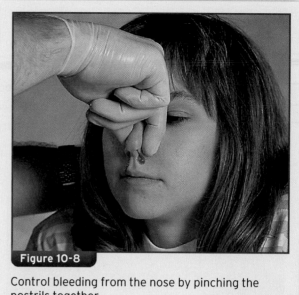

Figure 10-8

Control bleeding from the nose by pinching the nostrils together.

▶ Knocked-Out Tooth

A knocked-out tooth is a dental emergency **Figure 10-9**. For successful replantation of the tooth, it is important to locate the tooth and prevent it from becoming dried out, and to protect the ligament fibers on the roots from damage.

Care for a Knocked-Out Tooth

To care for a knocked-out tooth:
1. Place a rolled or folded gauze pad in the socket to control bleeding.
2. Handle the tooth by the crown, not the root.
3. Get the victim to a dentist promptly so the tooth can be successfully replaced in its socket. If more serious injuries exist, seek medical care.
4. The tooth should be kept moist. Several options exist:
   - If the victim is an adult and alert, the tooth can be laid inside the lower lip, between the teeth and lip.
   - If it is not possible to place the tooth in the mouth, have the victim spit into a cup, and place the tooth in the saliva.
   - If neither of the preceding options is possible, the tooth can be placed in whole milk or a saltwater solution (½ teaspoon salt in 1 quart of water). Use regular water if these options are not available.

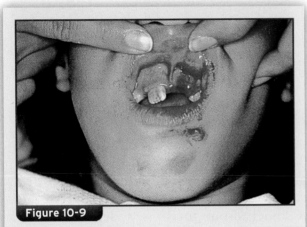

Figure 10-9

Tooth knocked out.

Spinal Injuries

Motor vehicle crashes, direct blows, falls from heights, physical assaults, and sports injuries are common causes of spinal injury. Suspect spine injuries in victims with significant head injuries, because the two are often associated.

Recognizing Spinal Injuries

The signs of spinal injuries include the following:
- Inability to move the limbs
- Numbness, tingling, weakness, or burning sensation in the limbs
- Deformity (odd-looking angle of the victim's head and neck)
- Neck or back pain

Care for Spinal Injuries

To care for a spinal injury:
1. Stabilize the head and neck to prevent movement **Figure 10-10**.
2. Check responsiveness and breathing. In case of vomiting, raise one arm above the head and roll the victim so the head rests on the raised arm.
3. Call 9-1-1.

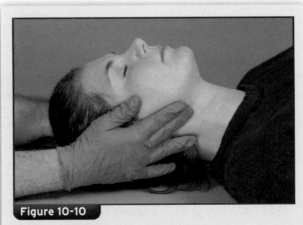

Figure 10-10

Prevent movement of the head and neck.

▶ Emergency Care Wrap-Up

Condition	What to Look For	What to Do
Scalp wound	• Scalp wound	1. Apply a sterile or clean dressing and direct pressure to control bleeding. 2. Keep head and shoulders raised. 3. Seek medical care.
Skull fracture	• Pain at point of injury • Deformity of the skull • Clear or bloody fluid draining from ears or nose • Heavy scalp bleeding • Penetrating wound	1. Check responsiveness and breathing and provide any necessary care. 2. Control bleeding by applying pressure around the edges of wound. 3. Stabilize the victim's head and neck against movement. 4. Call 9-1-1.
Brain injury (concussion)	• Befuddled facial expression (vacant stare) • Slownesss in answering questions • Unaware of surroundings or day of week • Slurred speech • Stumbling, inability to walk a straight line • Crying for no apparent reason • Inability to recite months of year in reverse order • Unresponsiveness • Headache, dizziness, and nausea • Repetitive speech	1. Check responsiveness and breathing and provide any necessary care. 2. Stabilize the victim's head and neck against movement. 3. Control any scalp bleeding. 4. Call 9-1-1.
Eye injuries	• Loose foreign object in eye	1. Look for object underneath both lids. 2. If seen, remove with wet gauze.
	• Penetrating eye injury	1. If object is still in eye, protect eye and stabilize long objects. 2. Call 9-1-1.
	• Blow to the eye	1. Apply an ice or cold pack. 2. Seek medical care if vision is affected.
	• Eye avulsion • Eyeball knocked out of its socket	1. Cover eye loosely with wet dressing. 2. DO NOT try to put eye back into socket. 3. Call 9-1-1.
	• Cuts of eye or lid	1. If eyeball is cut, DO NOT apply pressure. 2. If only eyelid is cut, apply dressing with gentle pressure. 3. Call 9-1-1.
	• Chemicals in eye	1. Flush with water for 20 minutes and loosely bandage with wet dressings. 2. Call 9-1-1.
	• Eye burns from light	1. Cover eyes with cold, wet dressings. 2. Seek medical care.

Nosebleeds	• Nosebleeds	1. Have victim sit and lean slightly forward.
		2. Pinch nose for 5 to 10 minutes.
		3. Seek medical care if:
		  • Bleeding does not stop
		  • Bleeding is associated with a broken nose

Broken nose	• Pain, swelling, and possibly crooked nose • Bleeding and breathing difficulty through nostrils • Black eyes appearing 1 to 2 days after injury	1. Care for nosebleed. 2. Apply an ice or cold pack. 3. Call 9-1-1.
Mouth injuries	• Bitten lip or tongue	1. Apply direct pressure. 2. Apply an ice or cold pack.
	• Knocked-out tooth	1. Control bleeding (place rolled gauze in socket). 2. Find tooth and preserve it in the victim's saliva, milk, or a saltwater solution. Handle the tooth by the crown, not the root. 3. See dentist as soon as possible.
	• Toothache	1. Rinse mouth and use dental floss to remove trapped food. 2. Seek dental care.
Spinal injuries	• Inability to move limbs • Numbness, tingling, weakness, or burning feeling in limbs • Deformity (head and neck at an odd angle) • Neck or back pain	1. Stabilize the head and neck against movement. 2. Check responsiveness and breathing and provide any necessary care. 3. Call 9-1-1.

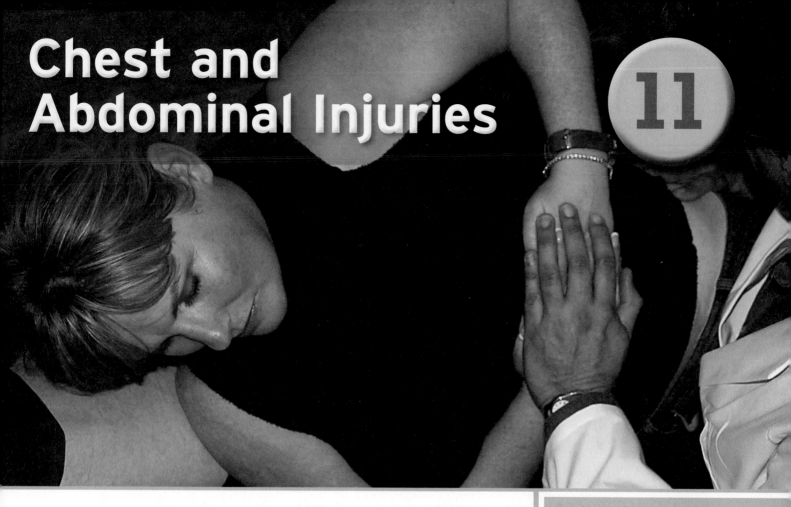

Chest and Abdominal Injuries

11

▶ Chest Injuries

Chest injuries can be closed or open. In a **closed chest injury**, the victim's skin is not broken. This type of injury is usually caused by blunt trauma. In an **open chest injury**, the skin has been broken and the chest wall is penetrated by an object such as a knife or bullet.

A responsive chest injury victim should usually sit up or, if the injury is on a side, be placed with the injured side down. This position prevents blood inside the chest cavity from seeping into the uninjured side and allows the uninjured side to expand.

closed chest injury
An injury to the chest in which the skin is not broken; usually due to blunt trauma.

open chest injury
An injury to the chest in which the chest wall itself is penetrated, either by a fractured rib or, more frequently, by an external object such as a bullet or knife.

Recognizing Rib Fractures

Rib fractures are a closed chest injury. The most common type of rib fracture is ribs fractured by a blow or a fall. A **flail chest** results when several ribs in the same area are broken in more than one place. The care for an isolated rib fracture and for flail chest is the same.

flail chest
A condition that occurs when several ribs in the same area are broken in more than one place.

Meeting ⊙SHA Recommendations

This chapter and the accompanying lesson cover the following *OSHA Best Practices Guide: Fundamentals of a Workplace First-Aid Program (2006)*:

4. Responding to Life-Threatening Emergencies
- Responding to Medical Emergencies
  - Chest pain;
  - Abdominal injury;
  - Impaled object

The signs of a rib fracture include:

- Sharp pain, especially when victim takes a deep breath, coughs, or moves
- Shallow breathing
- Victim holds the injured area, trying to reduce pain

Care for Rib Fractures

To care for a rib fracture:

1. Help the victim find the most comfortable resting position to make breathing easier.
2. Stabilize the ribs by having the victim hold a pillow or other similar soft object against the injured area, or use bandages to hold the pillow in place **Figure 11-1**.
3. Call 9-1-1.

Recognizing an Impaled Object

Impaled objects are open chest injuries where an object, such as a knife, is stuck in the chest.

Care for an Impaled Object

To care for an impaled object:

1. DO NOT remove object. Removing an embedded object can cause more damage.
2. Use bulky dressings or cloth to stabilize the object.
3. Call 9-1-1.

Recognizing a Sucking Chest Wound

A **sucking chest wound** results when a chest wound allows air to pass into and out of the chest cavity with each breath.

> **sucking chest wound**
> A chest wound that allows air to pass into and out of the chest cavity with each breath.

The signs of a sucking chest wound include:

- Blood bubbling out of a chest wound
- Sound of air being sucked into and out of the chest wound

Care for a Sucking Chest Wound

To care for a sucking chest wound:

1. Seal the wound with plastic or aluminum foil to stop air from entering the chest cavity. Tape three sides of the plastic or foil in place **Figure 11-2**. If neither item is available, you can use your gloved hand. This treatment prevents air from entering the chest but allows air to escape.
2. If the victim has trouble breathing or seems to be getting worse, remove the cover (or your hand) to let air escape, and then reapply.
3. Lay victim on the injured side.
4. Call 9-1-1.

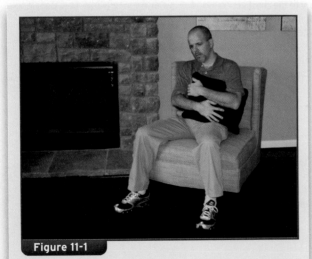

Figure 11-1

Stabilize chest with a soft object, such as a pillow, coat, or blanket (hold or tie).

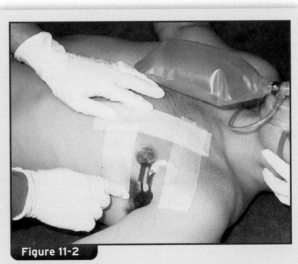

Figure 11-2

For a sucking chest wound, tape three sides of the plastic or foil in place.

▶ Abdominal Injuries

<u>**closed abdominal injuries**</u>
Injuries to the abdomen that occur as a result of a direct blow from a blunt object.

<u>**open abdominal injuries**</u>
Injuries to the abdomen that include penetrating wounds and protruding organs.

Abdominal injuries are either open or closed. <u>Closed abdominal injuries</u> occur as the result of a direct blow from a blunt object. <u>Open abdominal injuries</u> include penetrating wounds, impaled objects, and protruding organs. The risk of infection is high. An impaled object in the abdomen is cared for in the same manner as an embedded object in the chest: Stabilize the object and call 9-1-1.

Recognizing a Closed Abdominal Injury

The signs of a closed abdominal injury include bruises, pain, tenderness, and muscle tightness.

Care for a Closed Abdominal Injury

To care for a closed abdominal injury:
1. Place the victim in a comfortable position with the legs pulled up toward the abdomen.
2. Care for shock.
3. Call 9-1-1.

Recognizing a Protruding Organ

<u>**protruding organ injury**</u>
A severe injury to the abdomen in which the internal organs escape or protrude from the wound.

A <u>protruding organ injury</u> refers to a severe injury to the abdomen in which the internal organs escape or protrude from the wound.

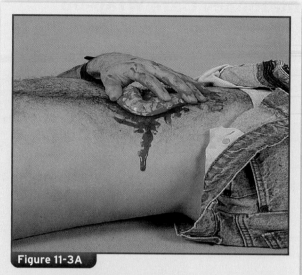

Figure 11-3A

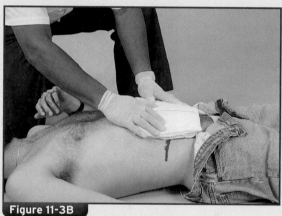

Figure 11-3B

Bandaging an open abdominal wound.
A. Open abdominal wounds are serious injuries.
B. Cover organs with a moist, sterile or clean dressing.

CAUTION

DO NOT try to reinsert protruding organs into the abdomen—you could introduce infection or damage the organs.

DO NOT cover the organs tightly.

Care for a Protruding Organ

To care for protruding organs:
1. Place the victim in a comfortable position with the knees bent and the legs pulled up toward the abdomen.
2. Cover protruding organs loosely with a moist, sterile or clean dressing. Do not use material that can come apart when wet, such as tissue. Clean plastic wrap or foil is a good choice if sterile gauze is not available **Figures 11-3A, B** .
3. Care for shock.
4. Call 9-1-1.

▶ Emergency Care Wrap-Up

Condition	What to Look For	What to Do
Rib fractures	• Sharp pain with deep breaths, coughing, or moving • Shallow breathing • Holding of injured area to reduce pain	1. Place victim in comfortable position. 2. Support ribs with a pillow, blanket, or coat (either holding or tying with bandages). 3. Call 9-1-1.
Impaled object	• Object remains in wound	1. DO NOT remove object from wound. 2. Use bulky dressings or cloths to stabilize the object. 3. Call 9-1-1.
Sucking chest wound	• Blood bubbling out of wound • Sound of air being sucked in and out of wound	1. Seal wound to stop air from entering chest; tape three sides of plastic or foil or use gloved hand. 2. Remove cover to let air escape if victim worsens or has trouble breathing and then reapply. 3. Call 9-1-1.
Blow to abdomen (closed)	• Bruise or other marks • Muscle tightness and rigidity	1. Place victim in comfortable position with legs pulled up toward the abdomen. 2. Care for shock. 3. Call 9-1-1.
Protruding organs (open)	• Internal organs escaping from abdominal wound	1. Place victim in a comfortable position with the legs pulled up toward the abdomen. 2. DO NOT reinsert organs into the abdomen. 3. Cover organs with a moist, sterile or clean dressing. 4. Care for shock. 5. Call 9-1-1.

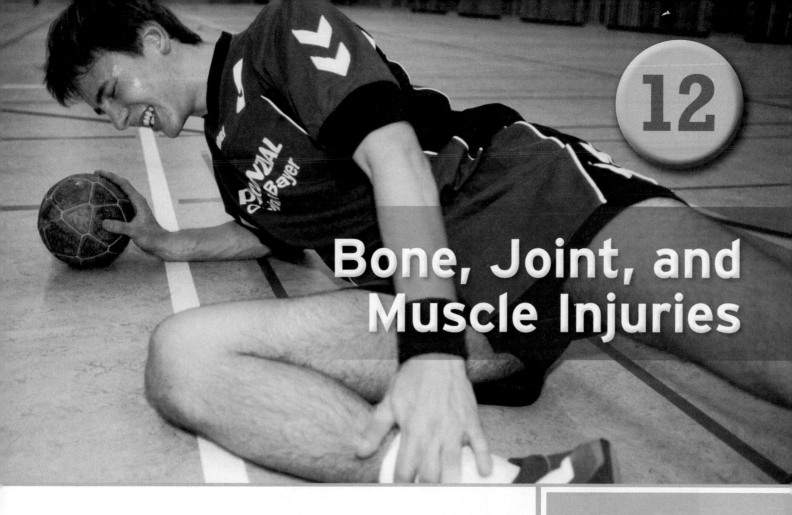

12

Bone, Joint, and Muscle Injuries

► Bone Injuries

A <u>fracture</u> is a break or crack in a bone. There are two categories of fractures (**Figure 12-1**):

- <u>Closed fracture:</u> No open wound exists around the fracture site (**Figure 12-2**).
- <u>Open fracture:</u> An open wound exists, and the broken bone end may be protruding through the skin (**Figure 12-3**).

fracture
Break in a bone.

closed fracture
A fracture with no open wound.

open fracture
A fracture with an open wound and possible protruding bone.

Recognizing Bone Injuries

It may be difficult to tell if a bone is broken. A good indication of a possible broken bone is the inability to use the injured part normally. The mnemonic DOTS can also be used to identify signs of a possible fracture:

- *D*eformity might not be obvious. Compare the injured part with the uninjured part on the other side.
- *O*pen wound may indicate an underlying fracture.
- *T*enderness and pain are commonly found only at the injury site. The victim can usually point to the site of the pain or feel pain when it is touched.
- *S*welling caused by bleeding happens rapidly after a fracture.

Meeting ◎SHA Recommendations

This chapter and the accompanying lesson cover the following *OSHA Best Practices Guide: Fundamentals of a Workplace First-Aid Program (2006)*:

5. **Responding to Non-Life-Threatening Emergencies**
   - Musculoskeletal Injuries
     – Fractures;
     – Sprains, strains, contusions and cramps.

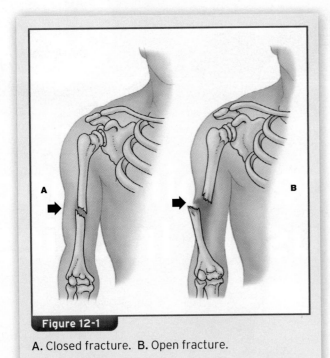

Figure 12-1

A. Closed fracture. B. Open fracture.

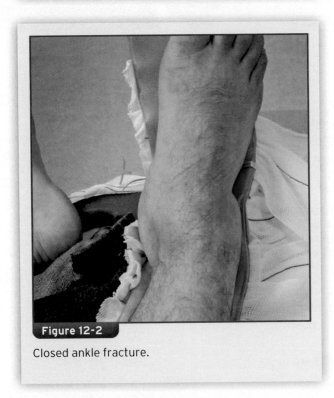

Figure 12-2

Closed ankle fracture.

Other indications of fracture can include:
- A grating or grinding sensation that can be felt and sometimes even heard when the ends of the broken bone rub together.
- The victim heard or felt the bone snap.

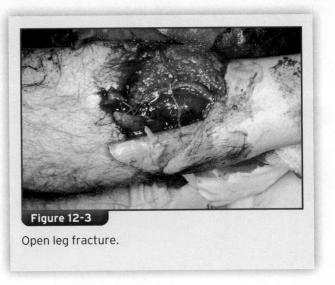

Figure 12-3

Open leg fracture.

Care for Bone Injuries

To care for a bone injury:
1. Allow the victim to support the injured area in the most comfortable position.
2. Stabilize the injured part to prevent movement.
   - If emergency medical services (EMS) will arrive soon, stabilize the injured part with your hands until they arrive.
   - If EMS will be delayed, or if you are taking the victim to medical care, stabilize the injured part with a **splint**.

> **splint**
> A device used to stabilize an injured extremity.

3. If the injury is an open fracture, do not push on any protruding bone. Cover the wound and exposed bone with a dressing.
4. Apply an ice or cold pack if possible to help reduce the swelling and pain.
5. Call 9-1-1 for any open fractures or large bone fractures (such as the thigh) or when transporting the victim would be difficult or would aggravate the injury.

▶ Splinting

A splint is a device that can be used to stabilize a bone or joint injury. Splinting an injured area helps reduce pain and prevent further damage to muscles, nerves, and blood vessels.

Types of Splints

A self-splint, or anatomic splint, is one in which the injured body part is tied to an uninjured part (for example, an injured finger to the adjacent finger, an injured arm to the chest, or the legs to each other) **Figure 12-4**.

A rigid splint is an inflexible device such as a padded board, a piece of heavy cardboard, or a commercially available moldable splint, such as a SAM splint, molded to fit the extremity. It must be long enough so that it can stabilize the area above and below the fracture site **Figure 12-5**.

A soft splint, such as a pillow or rolled blanket, is useful mainly for stabilizing fractures of the ankle and wrist **Figure 12-6**.

Applying a Splint

To apply a splint, follow the steps shown in **Skill Drills 12-1, 12-2, and 12-3**.

▶ Joint Injuries

sprain
Torn joint ligaments.

A **sprain** is a common injury to a joint in which the ligaments and other tissues are damaged by violent stretching or twisting. Attempts to move or use the joint increase the pain. Common locations for sprains include the ankles, wrists, and knees.

dislocation
Bone ends at a joint are no longer in contact.

A **dislocation** is a serious and less common joint injury. It occurs when a joint comes apart and stays apart, with the bone ends no longer in contact. The shoulders, elbows, fingers, hips, knees, and ankles are the joints most frequently dislocated.

Recognizing Joint Injuries

The signs of a sprain or dislocation are similar to those of a fracture: pain, swelling, and inability to use the injured joint normally. The main sign of a dislocation is deformity. Its appearance will be different from that of an uninjured joint **Figures 12-7A, B**.

Care for Joint Injuries

To care for a joint injury:
1. If you suspect a dislocation, apply a splint if EMS will be delayed. Provide care as you would for a fracture. Do not try to put the displaced part back into its normal position

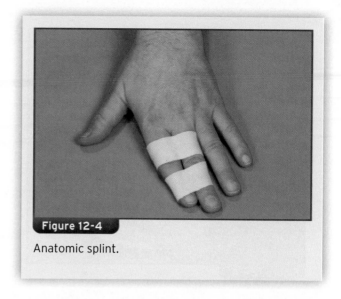
Figure 12-4
Anatomic splint.

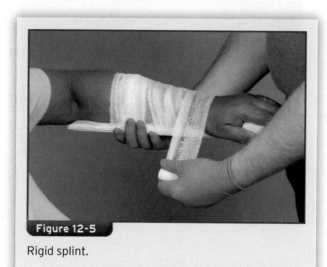
Figure 12-5
Rigid splint.

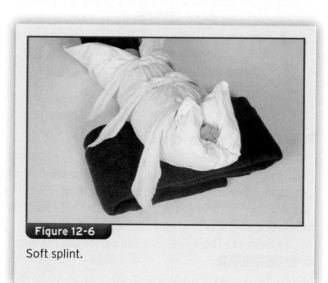
Figure 12-6
Soft splint.

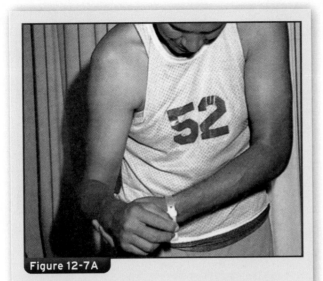

Figure 12-7A

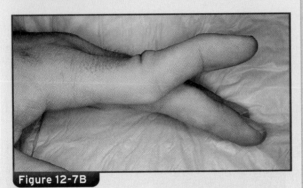

Figure 12-7B

A. Dislocated shoulder. B. Dislocated finger.

CAUTION

DO NOT apply an ice or cold pack for more than 30 minutes at a time.

DO NOT stop using an ice or cold pack too soon. A common mistake is the early use of heat, which increases circulation to the injured area, resulting in swelling and pain.

▶ Muscle Injuries

A muscle **strain**, also known as a muscle pull, occurs when a muscle is overstretched and tears. Back muscles are commonly strained when people lift heavy objects.

A muscle **contusion**, or bruise, results from a blow to the muscle. A muscle **cramp** occurs when a muscle goes into an uncontrolled spasm.

strain
Stretched or torn muscle.

contusion
A bruise; an injury that causes a hemorrhage in or beneath the skin but does not break the skin.

cramp
A painful spasm, usually of a muscle.

Recognizing Muscle Injuries

The signs of a muscle strain include the following:
- Sharp pain
- Tenderness when the area is touched
- Weakness and loss of function of the injured area
- Stiffness and pain when the victim moves the muscle

The signs of a muscle contusion include the following:
- Pain and tenderness
- Swelling
- Bruise appearing hours after the injury

The signs of a muscle cramp include the following:
- Spasm
- Pain
- Inability to use the injured area

Care for Muscle Injuries

Care for muscle strains and contusions includes resting the affected muscles and applying an ice or cold pack. To care for a muscle cramp, have the victim stretch the affected muscle or apply pressure directly to it.

because nerve and blood vessel damage could result.

2. If you suspect a sprain, use the RICE procedure (see Skill Drill 12-4).

3. Seek medical care. Call 9-1-1 for any dislocations or injuries for which transporting the victim would be difficult or would aggravate the injury.

▶ RICE Procedure

RICE is the acronym for rest, ice, compression, and elevation. This mnemonic will help you remember the care for a joint injury (such as a sprain) or a muscle injury (for example, a strain or contusion).

To perform the RICE procedure, follow the steps in Skill Drill 12-4 .

skill drill

12-1   Applying a Self (Anatomic) Splint: Upper or Lower Arm

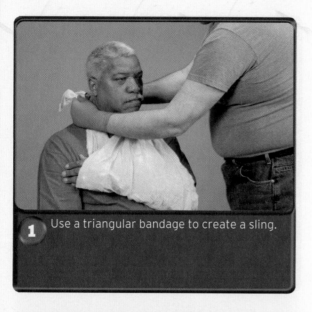

1 Use a triangular bandage to create a sling.

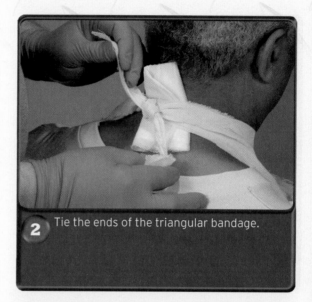

2 Tie the ends of the triangular bandage.

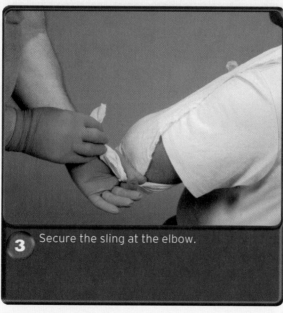

3 Secure the sling at the elbow.

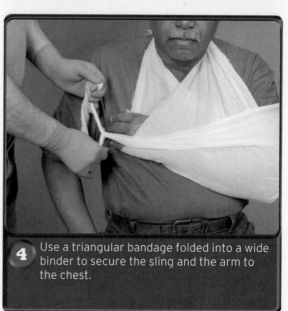

4 Use a triangular bandage folded into a wide binder to secure the sling and the arm to the chest.

skill drill

12-2   Applying a Rigid Splint: Lower Arm

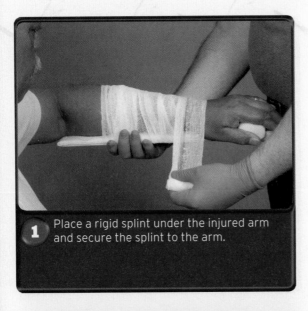

1 Place a rigid splint under the injured arm and secure the splint to the arm.

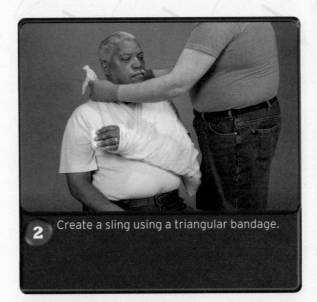

2 Create a sling using a triangular bandage.

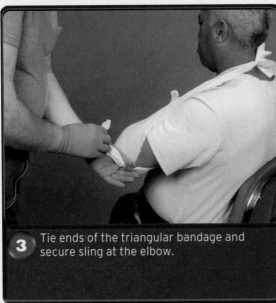

3 Tie ends of the triangular bandage and secure sling at the elbow.

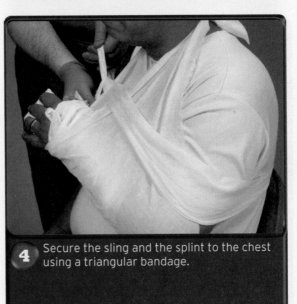

4 Secure the sling and the splint to the chest using a triangular bandage.

skill drill

12-3   Applying a Soft Splint: Lower Arm

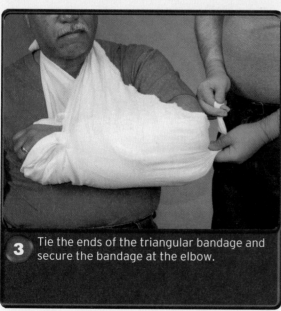

1 Place a soft splint around the injured area and secure the splint with several triangular bandages folded into binders.

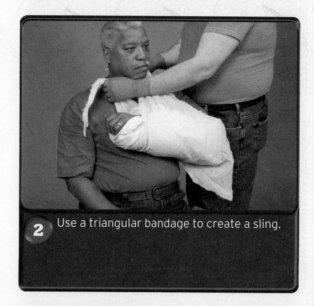

2 Use a triangular bandage to create a sling.

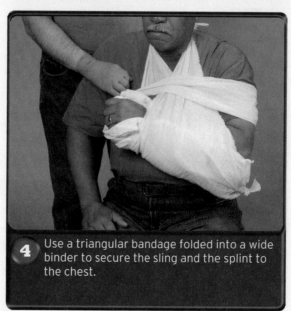

3 Tie the ends of the triangular bandage and secure the bandage at the elbow.

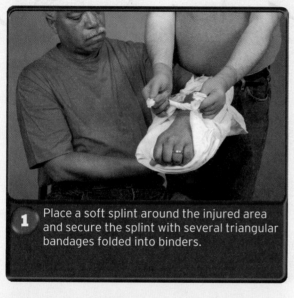

4 Use a triangular bandage folded into a wide binder to secure the sling and the splint to the chest.

skill drill

12-4   RICE Procedure

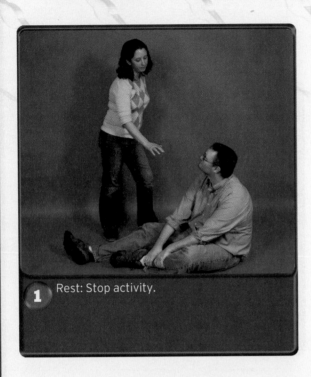

1 Rest: Stop activity.

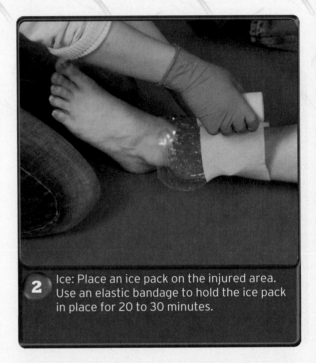

2 Ice: Place an ice pack on the injured area. Use an elastic bandage to hold the ice pack in place for 20 to 30 minutes.

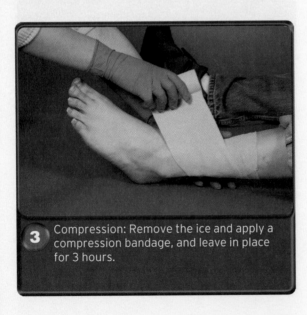

3 Compression: Remove the ice and apply a compression bandage, and leave in place for 3 hours.

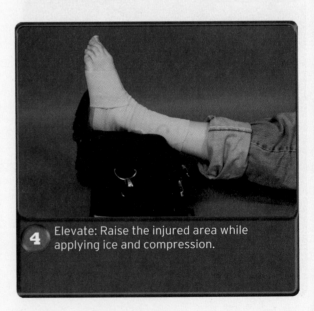

4 Elevate: Raise the injured area while applying ice and compression.

▶ Emergency Care Wrap-Up

Condition	What to Look For	What to Do
Fractures (broken bones)	• DOTS (deformity, open wound, tenderness, swelling) • Inability to use injured part normally • Grating or grinding sensation felt or heard • Victim heard or felt bone snap	1. Bandage any open wound. 2. Splint the injured area. 3. Apply ice or cold pack. 4. Seek medical care: Depending on the severity, call 9-1-1 or transport to medical care.
Dislocation or sprain (joint injury)	• Deformity • Pain • Swelling • Inability to use injured part normally	Dislocation 1. Splint the injured area. 2. Apply ice or cold pack. 3. Call 9-1-1. Sprain 1. Use RICE procedures.
Strain (muscle injury)	• Sharp pain • Tenderness when area is touched • Weaknesss and loss of function of injured area • Stiffness and pain when victim moves the muscle	1. Use RICE procedures.
Contusion (muscle injury)	• Pain and tenderness • Swelling • Bruise on injured area	1. Use RICE procedures.
Cramp (muscle injury)	• Spasm • Pain • Restriction or loss of movement	1. Stretch and/or apply direct pressure to the affected muscle.

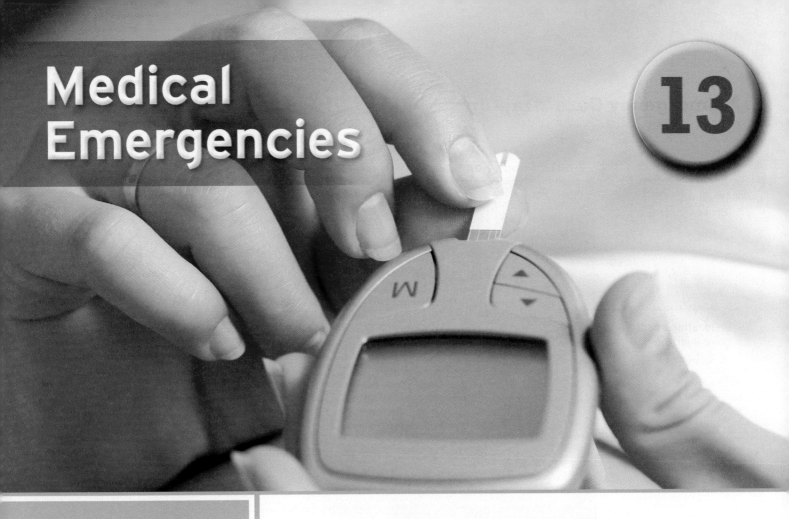

Medical Emergencies

13

Meeting OSHA Recommendations

This chapter and the accompanying lesson cover the following *OSHA Best Practices Guide: Fundamentals of a Workplace First-Aid Program (2006)*:

4. Responding to Life-Threatening Emergencies

- Assessing and treating a victim who has an unexplained change in level of consciousness

- Responding to Medical Emergencies
  - Chest pain;
  - Breathing problems;
  - Hypoglycemia in diabetics taking insulin;
  - Seizures;
  - Pregnancy complications;
  - Reduced level of consciousness.

▶ Changes in Consciousness

Victims can be conscious (responsive), or unconscious (unresponsive). Not all victims are fully alert, and some may only respond to different levels of stimulation. Some may respond to your voice, whereas others only respond to physical stimulation (for example, squeezing the hand or shoulder muscle). The level of consciousness indicates how well the brain is functioning.

What to Look For

The mnemonic STOP offers clues when you notice changes in consciousness and you are not sure what is causing it ⬤ Table 13-1 .

What to Do

1. Perform a primary and secondary check and provide care as needed.
2. If unresponsive and not breathing, perform CPR.
3. If unresponsive and vomiting, roll the victim onto his or her side.
4. Call 9-1-1.

74

Table 13-1 Changes in Consciousness

S = Sugar, Seizures, Stroke, Shock	Blood glucose (sugar) too low (for example, in an insulin reaction)
T = Temperature	Too high (heatstroke) or too low (hypothermia)
O = Oxygen	Inadequate oxygen
P = Poisoning or pressure on brain	Drug/alcohol overdose, carbon monoxide poisoning, head injury

▶ Chest Pain

Chest pain can signal a heart attack, but there are other causes and not all of them involve the heart.

Heart Attack

A heart attack occurs when the oxygen-rich blood supply to part of the heart is blocked. Pain comes from a lack of oxygen to the heart muscle. The chest pain can be crushing, vice-like, and squeezing and typically lasts more than 10 minutes. It may spread to the jaw or down the arms, usually the left.

To care for chest pain associated with a heart attack:
1. Call 9-1-1.
2. Have the victim rest.
3. If the victim has physician-prescribed nitroglycerin, help him or her take it (usually a small tablet or spray placed under the tongue).
4. If the victim is not allergic to aspirin, give four chewable aspirin tablets (81 mg each) or one regular aspirin tablet (325 mg).

Respiratory Infection

Pneumonia, bronchitis, or pleurisy can cause chest pain, as well as a cough, fever, sore throat, and production of saliva. Seek medical care for respiratory infections.

Muscle Pain

Physical activity and overexertion can result in chest pain. Rest and an over-the-counter pain medication are usually all that are needed to provide relief.

▶ Breathing Difficulty

Breathing difficulty can result from injuries to the chest or head and from illnesses such as heart attack, anaphylaxis, or asthma. Asthma is a condition in which air passages narrow and mucus builds up, resulting in poor oxygen exchange. It can be triggered by such things as an allergy, cold exposure, and smoke. Hyperventilation is fast breathing, which can be caused by emotional stress, anxiety, and medical conditions.

asthma
An acute spasm of the smaller air passages that causes difficult breathing and wheezing.

hyperventilation
Abnormally fast breathing.

Recognizing Breathing Difficulty

The signs of breathing difficulty include the following:
- Breathing that is abnormally fast or slow
- Breathing that is abnormally deep (gasping) or shallow
- Noisy breathing, including wheezing (seen with asthma) or gurgling, crowing, or snoring sounds
- Bluish lips
- Need to pause while speaking to catch breath

Care for Breathing Difficulty

To care for a victim with breathing difficulty:
1. Help the victim into the most comfortable position. This is often seated upright.
2. Call 9-1-1.
3. If the victim has a prescribed asthma inhaler, assist the victim in using it Figure 13-1.
4. If the victim is hyperventilating (breathing fast) due to anxiety, have him or her inhale through the nose, hold the breath for several seconds, then exhale slowly.

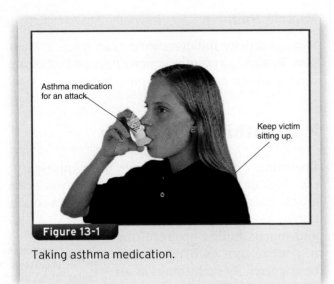

Figure 13-1

Taking asthma medication.

Asthma medication for an attack.

Keep victim sitting up.

▶ Fainting

Fainting can happen suddenly when blood flow to the brain is interrupted. Causes include exhaustion, lack of food, reaction to pain or the sight of blood, hearing bad news, standing too long without moving, or problems with the heart.

Recognizing Fainting

The signs of fainting include the following:
- Sudden, brief unresponsiveness
- Pale skin
- Sweating

Care for Fainting

To care for fainting:
1. Check responsiveness and breathing and provide care as needed.
2. Loosen any restrictive clothing.
3. If the victim fell, check for injuries.
4. Most fainting episodes in younger patients are not serious, and the victim recovers quickly. Seek medical care if the victim:
   - Has repeated fainting episodes
   - Does not quickly become responsive
   - Becomes unresponsive while sitting or lying down
   - Faints for no apparent reason
   - Is elderly

▶ Seizures

A <u>seizure</u> results from an abnormal stimulation of the brain's cells. A variety of causes can lead to seizures, including the following:
- Epilepsy
- Heatstroke
- Poisoning
- Electric shock
- Hypoglycemia
- High fever
- Brain injury, tumor, or stroke
- Alcohol or other drug withdrawal or abuse

> **seizure**
> Sudden violent muscle rigidity and jerky movements (convulsions) resulting from abnormal stimulation of the brain's cells.

Recognizing a Seizure

The signs of a seizure will vary depending on the type of seizure and can include the following:
- Sudden falling
- Unresponsiveness
- Rigid body and arching of the back
- Jerky muscle movement

Care for a Seizure

To care for a victim having a seizure:
1. Prevent injury by moving away any dangerous objects.
2. Loosen any restrictive clothing.
3. Roll the victim onto his or her side to help keep the airway clear.
4. Call 9-1-1 for seizures occurring for no known reason.

▶ Diabetic Emergencies

<u>Diabetes</u> results when the body fails to produce sufficient amounts of insulin, which helps regulate blood glucose level.

> **diabetes**
> A disease in which the body is unable to use glucose normally because of a deficiency or total lack of insulin.

There are two types of diabetes:
- *Type 1:* People with type 1 diabetes require external (not made by the body) insulin to allow glucose to pass from the blood into cells.
- *Type 2:* People with type 2 diabetes may not be dependent on external insulin to allow glucose into cells and may take only oral medication to help control the disease.

The body is continuously balancing glucose and insulin. Too much insulin and not enough glucose leads to low blood glucose (hypoglycemia). Too much glucose and not enough insulin leads to high blood glucose (hyperglycemia) **Figure 13-2** .

Recognizing Low Blood Glucose

hypoglycemia
Abnormally low blood glucose level.

A very low blood glucose level, called **hypoglycemia**, can be caused by too much insulin, too little or delayed food intake, exercise, illness, or any combination of these factors.

In a person with diabetes, the signs of low blood glucose include the following:

- Sudden onset of symptoms
- Staggering, poor coordination
- Anger, bad temper
- Pale skin
- Confusion, disorientation
- Sudden hunger
- Excessive sweating
- Trembling
- Seizure
- Unresponsiveness

Care for Low Blood Glucose

To care for a diabetic with low blood glucose (hypoglycemia) who is responsive and can swallow:

1. Give sugar, such as one tablespoon, half a can of soda, juice, three glucose tablets, or one tube of glucose gel **Figure 13-3** .
2. If there is no improvement, call 9-1-1.

If the victim is unresponsive, do not give anything by mouth. Call 9-1-1.

Recognizing High Blood Glucose

hyperglycemia
Abnormally high blood glucose level.

Hyperglycemia is the opposite of hypoglycemia. Hyperglycemia occurs when the body has too much glucose in the blood but is unable to get it to the cells. This condition may be caused by insufficient insulin, overeating, inactivity, illness, stress, or a combination of these factors.

In a person with diabetes, there may be no signs of high blood glucose initially. Signs of high blood glucose requiring medical attention may include:

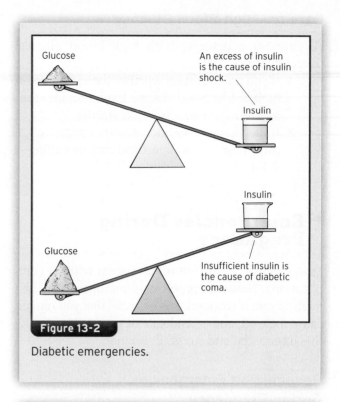

Figure 13-2
Diabetic emergencies.

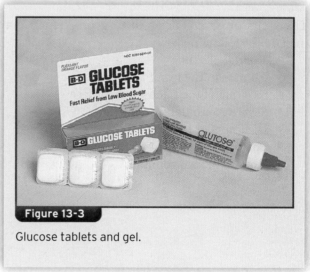

Figure 13-3
Glucose tablets and gel.

- Gradual onset of symptoms
- Drowsiness
- Extreme thirst
- Very frequent urination
- Warm and dry skin
- Vomiting
- Fruity, sweet breath odor
- Rapid breathing
- Unresponsiveness

Care for High Blood Glucose

To care for a diabetic with high blood glucose (hyperglycemia):

1. If you are uncertain whether the victim has a high or low blood glucose level, provide care as you would for low blood glucose.
2. If the victim's condition does not improve in 15 minutes, seek medical care by calling 9-1-1.

▶ Emergencies During Pregnancy

Most pregnancies are normal and occur without complications. However, problems sometimes arise, and medical care is required. It is essential that you remain calm, focused, and considerate of the mother during this unforeseen and stressful situation.

Recognizing Emergencies During Pregnancy

The signs of emergencies during pregnancy may include the following:

- Vaginal bleeding
- Cramps in the lower abdomen
- Swelling of the hands, feet, or face
- Severe continuous headache
- Dizziness or fainting
- Blurring of vision or seeing spots
- Uncontrollable vomiting

Care for Pregnancy Emergencies

If the victim is experiencing vaginal bleeding or abdominal pain or injury:

1. Keep her warm and on her left side.
2. If vaginal bleeding is present, have the victim place a sanitary napkin or any sterile or clean pad over the opening of the vagina.
3. Save any blood-soaked pads and all tissues that are passed. Send this with the woman when she is transported for medical care.
4. Seek medical care.

▶ Emergency Care Wrap-Up

Condition	What to Look For	What to Do
Heart attack	• Chest pressure, squeezing, or pain • Pain spreading to shoulders, neck, jaw, or arms • Dizziness, sweating, nausea • Shortness of breath	1. Help victim take his or her prescribed medication. 2. Call 9-1-1. 3. Help victim into a comfortable position. 4. Give four chewable aspirin (81 mg each) or one regular aspirin (325 mg).
Breathing difficulty	• Abnormally fast or slow breathing • Abnormally deep or shallow breathing • Noisy breathing • Bluish lips • Need to pause while speaking to catch breath	**Unknown reason** 1. Help victim into a comfortable position. 2. Call 9-1-1. **Asthma attack** 1. Help victim into a comfortable position. 2. Help victim use inhaler. 3. Call 9-1-1 if victim does not improve. **Hyperventilating** 1. Encourage victim to inhale, hold breath a few seconds, then exhale. 2. Call 9-1-1 if condition does not improve.
Fainting	• Sudden, brief unresponsiveness • Pale skin • Sweating	1. Check responsiveness and breathing. 2. Check for injuries if victim fell. 3. Call 9-1-1 if needed.
Seizures	• Sudden falling • Unresponsiveness • Rigid body and arching of back • Jerky muscle movement	1. Prevent injury. 2. Loosen any tight clothing. 3. Roll victim onto his or her side. 4. Call 9-1-1 if needed.
Diabetic emergencies	**Low blood glucose** • Develops very quickly • Anger, bad temper • Hunger • Pale, sweaty skin • Confusion **High blood glucose** • Develops gradually • Thirst • Frequent urination • Fruity, sweet breath odor • Warm and dry skin	1. If uncertain about high or low glucose level, give sugar if the victim is able to take the sugar by mouth. 2. Call 9-1-1 if conditions do not improve within 15 minutes.
Pregnancy emergencies	• Vaginal bleeding • Cramps in lower abdomen • Swelling of face or fingers • Severe continuous headache • Dizziness or fainting • Blurring of vision or seeing spots • Uncontrollable vomiting	**Vaginal bleeding or abdominal pain or injury** 1. Keep victim warm. 2. For vaginal bleeding, place sanitary napkin or sterile or clean pad over opening of vagina. 3. Send blood-soaked pad and tissues with victim to medical care. 4. Seek medical care.

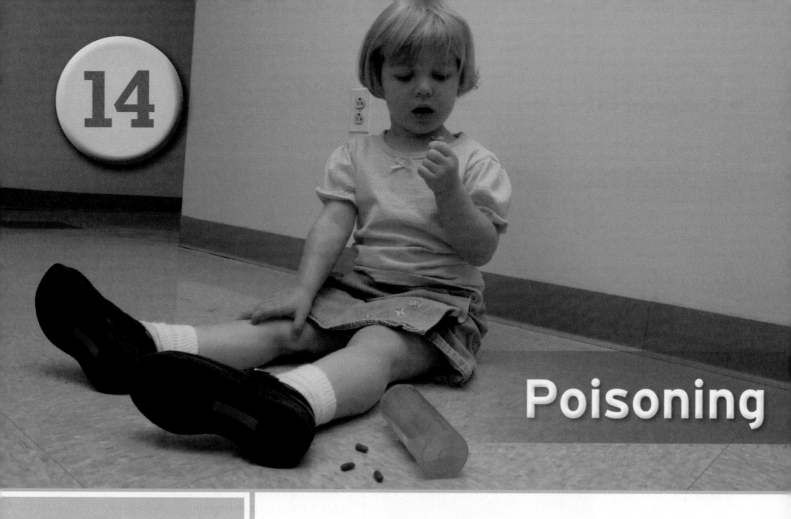

14

Poisoning

Meeting OSHA Recommendations

This chapter and the accompanying lesson cover the following *OSHA Best Practices Guide: Fundamentals of a Workplace First-Aid Program (2006)*:

4. Responding to Life-Threatening Emergencies

- Poisoning

  - Ingested poisons: alkali, acid, and systemic poisons. Role of the Poison Control Center (1-800-222-1222);

  - Inhaled poisons: carbon monoxide; hydrogen sulfide; smoke; and other chemical fumes, vapors, and gases. Assessing the toxic potential of the environment and the need for respirators;

  - Knowledge of the chemicals at the worksite and of first aid and treatment for inhalation or ingestion;

  - Effects of alcohol and illicit drugs so that the first aid provider can recognize the physiologic and behavioral effects of these substances.

▶ Poisons

poison
Any substance that impairs health or causes death by its chemical action when it enters the body or comes in contact with the skin; also known as a toxin.

A **poison** (also known as a *toxin*) is any substance that impairs health or causes death by its chemical action when it enters the body or comes in contact with the skin.

▶ Ingested Poisons

ingested poisoning
Poisoning caused by swallowing a toxic substance.

Ingested poisoning occurs when the victim swallows a toxic substance. Fortunately, most poisons have little toxic effect or are ingested in such small amounts that severe poisoning rarely occurs. However, the potential for severe or fatal poisoning is always present. About 80% of all poisonings happen by ingesting a toxic substance.

Recognizing Ingested Poisoning

The signs of ingested poisoning include the following:

- Abdominal pain and cramping
- Nausea or vomiting
- Diarrhea
- Burns, odor, or stains around and in the mouth
- Drowsiness or unresponsiveness
- Poison container nearby

Care for Ingested Poisons

To care for victims who have ingested poisons:

1. Determine the following:
   - The age and size of the victim
   - What was swallowed (read container label; save vomit for analysis)
   - How much was swallowed (for example, a dozen tablets)
   - When it was swallowed

2. For a responsive victim, call the poison control center at 1-800-222-1222. Most poisonings can be treated by following the instructions received by telephone from a **poison control center**. The poison control center may advise you to dilute the poison, induce vomiting, or provide **activated charcoal** if available. The poison control center staff will also advise you if a call to 9-1-1 or additional medical care are needed.

3. Call 9-1-1 for an unresponsive and breathing victim. Provide CPR if the victim is unresponsive and not breathing until EMS personnel arrive.

> **poison control center**
> Medical facility providing immediate, free, expert advice anytime by calling 1-800-222-1222.
>
> **activated charcoal**
> Powdered charcoal that has been treated to increase its powers of absorption. Used to treat patients who have ingested poisons.

▶ Alcohol and Other Drug Emergencies

Poisoning caused by an overdose or abuse of medications and other substances, including alcohol, is common. The most commonly abused drug in the United States is alcohol.

Recognizing Alcohol Intoxication

Helping an intoxicated person can be difficult because the person may be belligerent or combative. The victim's condition may be quite serious, even life threatening. Although the following signs indicate alcohol intoxication, some can also mean injury or illness other than alcohol intoxication, such as diabetes:

- The odor of alcohol on a person's breath or clothing
- Unsteadiness, staggering
- Confusion
- Slurred speech
- Nausea and vomiting
- Flushed face

FYI

Activated Charcoal

Activated charcoal is a fine, black, odorless powder that is available as a liquid. Activated charcoal prevents the absorption of most poisons and drugs by the stomach and intestines **Figure 14-1**.

Activated charcoal does not absorb all drugs well. Acids and alkalis (for example, bleach and ammonia), potassium, iron, alcohol, methanol, kerosene, gasoline, and cyanide require different treatment.

A drawback of activated charcoal is its grittiness and its appearance. Trying to improve the taste or consistency by adding chocolate syrup, sherbet, ice cream, or milk only decreases the charcoal's binding capacity.

CAUTION

DO NOT give water or milk to dilute poisons unless instructed to do so by a poison control center.

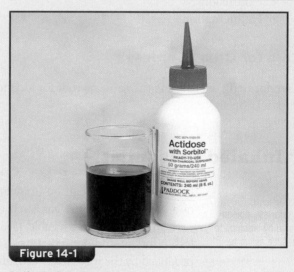

Figure 14-1

Activated charcoal.

Care for Alcohol Intoxication

To care for alcohol intoxication:

1. If the victim is responsive:
   - Check breathing.
   - Call the poison control center for advice (1-800-222-1222).
   - If the victim becomes violent, leave the area and call 9-1-1.

2. If the victim is unresponsive and breathing, then roll the victim to his or her side (recovery position). Call 9-1-1. If the victim is unresponsive and not breathing, begin CPR.

CAUTION

DO NOT let an intoxicated person sleep on his or her back.

DO NOT leave an intoxicated person alone, unless he or she becomes violent.

DO NOT try to handle a hostile intoxicated person by yourself.

Recognizing Drug Overdose

The condition of a person suffering from a drug overdose may be quite serious, even life threatening. The signs of drug overdose include the following:

- Drowsiness, anxiety, agitation, or hyperactivity
- Change in pupil size
- Confusion
- Hallucinations

Care for Drug Overdose

Care for drug overdose is the same as that for alcohol intoxication.

▶ Inhaled Poisoning

carbon monoxide
A colorless, odorless, poisonous gas formed by incomplete combustion, such as in fire.

Poisoning victims can be unaware of a gas's presence. A gas such as **carbon monoxide** is invisible, tasteless, odorless, and nonirritating. It is produced by the incomplete burning of organic material such as gasoline, wood, paper, charcoal, coal, and natural gas.

Recognizing Inhaled Poisoning

The signs of inhaled poisoning include the following:
- Headache
- Breathing difficulty
- Chest pain
- Nausea and vomiting

- Dizziness and visual changes (blurred or double vision)
- Unresponsiveness

Care for Inhaled Poisoning

To care for victims of inhaled poisons:
1. Get the victim out of the toxic environment and into fresh air.
2. Check responsiveness and breathing and provide care as needed.
3. Call 9-1-1.
4. Try to determine what substance was involved.

▶ Chemical Safety at the Worksite

To ensure chemical safety at the worksite, information must be available about the identities and hazards of the chemicals. OSHA's Hazard Communication Standard (HCS) requires the development and dissemination of such information:

- Chemical manufacturers and importers are required to evaluate the hazards of the chemicals they produce or import, and prepare labels and **Material Safety Data Sheets (MSDSs)** to convey the hazard information to their downstream customers.

Material Safety Data Sheet (MSDS)
Lists the hazardous ingredients of products, as well as their characteristics, effects on human health, and treatment for exposure.

- All employers with hazardous chemicals in their workplaces must have labels and MSDSs for their exposed workers and train them to handle the chemicals appropriately.

FYI

Material Safety Data Sheets

For each hazardous chemical in the workplace, an employer is required by law to maintain a copy of the MSDS. An MSDS lists the hazardous ingredients of a product, its physical and chemical characteristics, effects on human health, the chemicals with which it can react adversely, handling precautions, measures that can be used to control exposure and contain a spill, and emergency and first aid procedures.

▶ Plant Poisoning

More than 60 plants can cause allergic reactions, but poison ivy, poison oak, and poison sumac are by far the most common Figure 14-2A–C .

Recognizing Plant Poisoning

An allergic reaction usually occurs 24 to 72 hours after contact.

The signs of plant poisoning include the following:
- Rash Figure 14-3
- Itching
- Redness
- Blisters
- Swelling

Care for Plant Poisoning

To care for plant poisoning:
1. If available, put on medical exam gloves to avoid exposure to the plant oil. Wash the affected area with soap and water as soon as possible to remove oily resin.
2. For a mild reaction, have the victim do any of the following:
   - Soak in a lukewarm bath sprinkled with 1 to 2 cups of colloidal oatmeal (such as Aveeno)
   - Apply calamine lotion (calamine ointment if the skin becomes dry and cracked)
3. For a more severe reaction, care for the skin as you would for a mild reaction and seek medical care. A prescribed oral **corticosteroid** may be needed.

corticosteroid
Medication to lessen inflammation and relieve irritation.

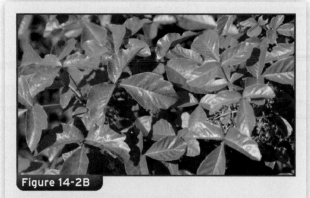

Figure 14-2B

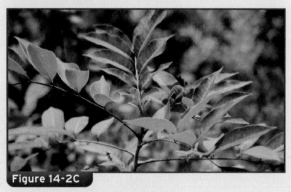

Figure 14-2C

Poisonous plants. **B.** Poison oak. **C.** Poison sumac.

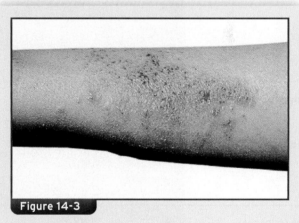

Figure 14-3
Poison ivy rash.

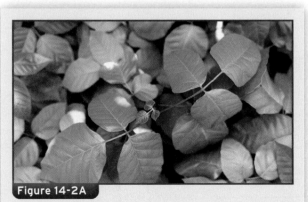

Figure 14-2A
Poisonous plants. **A.** Poison ivy.

▶ Emergency Care Wrap-Up

Condition	What to Look For	What to Do
Ingested (swallowed) poisoning	• Abdominal pain and cramping • Nausea or vomiting • Diarrhea • Burns, odor, or stains around and in mouth • Drowsiness or unresponsiveness • Poison container nearby	1. If the victim is responsive, call the poison control center at 1-800-222-1222 and follow the advice given. 2. If the victim is unresponsive, call 9-1-1. Place the victim on his or her side if breathing. If not breathing, start CPR.
Alcohol intoxication	• Alcohol odor on breath or clothing • Unsteadiness, staggering • Confusion • Slurred speech • Nausea and vomiting • Flushed face	1. If the victim is responsive: • Check breathing. • Call the poison control center for advice (1-800-222-1222). • If the victim becomes violent, leave area and call 9-1-1. 2. If the victim is unresponsive and breathing, roll the victim to his or her side (recovery position). Call 9-1-1. If the victim is unresponsive and not breathing, begin CPR.
Drug overdose	• Drowsiness, agitation, anxiety, hyperactivity • Change in pupil size • Confusion • Hallucinations	1. If the victim is responsive: • Check breathing. • Call the poison control center for advice (1-800-222-1222). • If the victim becomes violent, leave area and call 9-1-1. 2. If the victim is unresponsive and breathing, roll the victim to his or her side (recovery position). Call 9-1-1. If the victim is unresponsive and not breathing, begin CPR.
Inhaled poisoning	• Headache • Difficult breathing • Chest pain • Nausea and vomiting • Dizziness and vision difficulties • Unresponsiveness	1. Move victim to fresh air. 2. Check responsiveness and breathing and provide care as needed. 3. Call 9-1-1. 4. Try to determine what substance was involved.
Plant (contact) poisoning	• Rash • Itching • Redness • Blisters • Swelling	1. Wash with soap and water. 2. For mild reaction, use one of these: • 1–2 cups of colloidal oatmeal in bathwater • Calamine lotion 3. For severe reactions, perform step 2 and seek medical care.

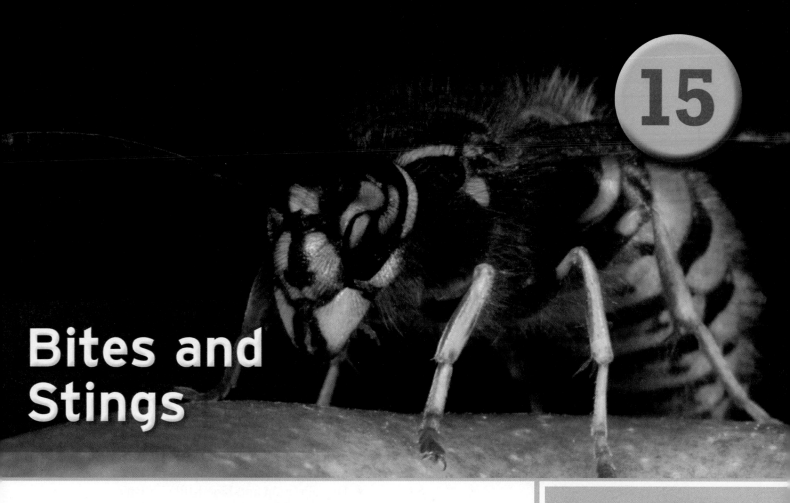

15

Bites and Stings

▶ Animal and Human Bites

An estimated one of every two Americans will be bitten by an animal or by another person. Dogs account for about 80% of all animal-bite injuries ◖ **Figure 15-1** ◗.

The human mouth contains a wide range of bacteria, so there is a chance that a wound caused by a human bite may become infected.

Rabies

<u>Rabies</u> is caused by a virus found in warm-blooded animals that spreads from one animal to another in the saliva, usually through a bite or scraping of the teeth against the skin.

> **rabies**
> An acute viral infection of the central nervous system transmitted by the bite of an infected animal.

An animal should be considered possibly rabid if:

- The animal attacked without provocation.
- The animal acted strangely or out of character (for example, a usually friendly dog is aggressive or a wild fox seems docile and "friendly").
- The animal was a high-risk species (for example, skunk, raccoon, or bat).

Report animal bites to the police or animal control officers; they should be the ones to capture the animal for observation. If the victim was bitten by a healthy domestic dog or cat, the animal should be confined and observed for 10 days for any illness.

Meeting ◎SHA Recommendations

This chapter and the accompanying lesson cover the following *OSHA Best Practices Guide: Fundamentals of a Workplace First-Aid Program (2006)*:

5. Responding to Non-Life-Threatening Emergencies

- Bites and Stings
  - Human and animal bites;
  - Bites and stings from insects; instruction in first aid treatment of anaphylactic shock.

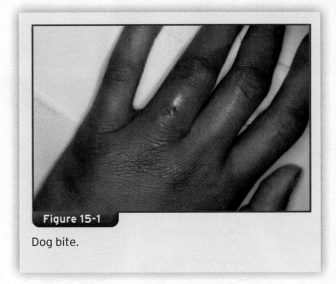

Figure 15-1

Dog bite.

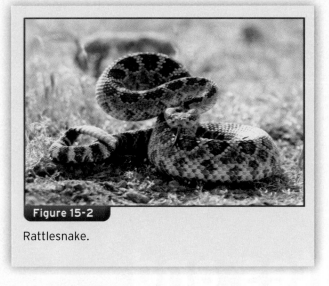

Figure 15-2

Rattlesnake.

If the victim was bitten by a wild animal, the incident should be considered a possible rabies exposure and medical care should be sought immediately. If a bat is found in a bedroom upon waking or in the room of an infant, child, person with disabilities, or an elderly person, then seek medical care immediately.

Care for an Animal or Human Bite

To care for an animal or human bite:

1. If the wound is not bleeding heavily, wash it with soap and water under pressure.
2. Flush the wound thoroughly with running water.
3. Control bleeding and cover the wound with a sterile or clean dressing.
4. Seek medical care for further wound cleaning and closure, and possible tetanus or rabies care.

▶ Snake Bites

Only four native snake species in the United States are venomous: rattlesnakes, copperheads, water moccasins (also known as cottonmouths), and coral snakes. Rattlesnakes **Figure 15-2**, copperheads, and water moccasins are pit vipers. The coral snake is small and colorful, with a black snout and a series of bright red, yellow, and black bands around its body (every other band is yellow). Venomous snakes from other countries also pose a snake-bite problem.

Recognizing a Venomous Snake Bite

The signs of a pit viper bite include the following:

- Severe, burning pain
- Puncture wounds about ½ to 1½ inches apart **Figure 15-3**
- Swelling
- Discoloration and blood-filled blisters possibly developing hours after the bite **Figure 15-4**
- Nausea, vomiting, sweating, and weakness

Care for a Venomous Snake Bite

To care for a pit viper bite:

1. Get the victim and bystanders away from the snake.
2. Keep the victim calm and limit movement. Immobilize the affected limb.
3. Gently wash the bitten area with soap and water. Do not attempt to trap or kill the snake.
4. If the bite is from a coral snake, apply mild pressure (able to slip a finger under it) by wrapping an elastic bandage (for example, an ACE bandage) over the bite site and the entire length of an arm or leg.
5. Seek medical care immediately.

CAUTION

DO NOT cut the victim's skin, attempt to suck out the venom, or apply ice or cold to the bitten area.

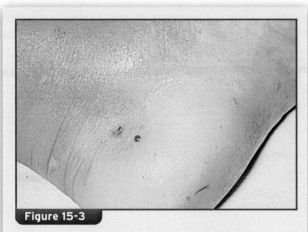

Figure 15-3

Rattlesnake bite (note the two fang marks).

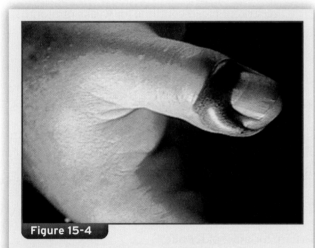

Figure 15-4

Copperhead bite 2 hours after bite.

FYI

Antivenin

Identifying the type of pit viper is not very important because the same antivenin is used to counteract all North American pit viper venom. However the antivenin for a coral snake is different.

antivenin
An antiserum containing antibodies against reptile or insect venom.

▶ Insect Stings

anaphylaxis
A severe allergic reaction that can be life threatening.

Most people will only experience the mild effects of an insect sting. However, some people can have severe allergic reactions (**anaphylaxis**).

Recognizing an Insect Sting

A rule of thumb is that the sooner symptoms develop after a sting, the more serious the reaction will be. Common signs of an insect sting are as follows:

- Pain
- Itching
- Swelling

Signs of a severe allergic reaction (anaphylaxis) include:

- Difficulty breathing
- Tightness in the chest
- Swelling of the tongue, mouth, or throat
- Dizziness and nausea

Care for an Insect Sting

To care for an insect sting:

1. If the stinger is embedded, remove it as quickly as possible using any removal method (e.g., brush it away with your hand, scrape it with a fingernail, or scrape it with a hard object such as a credit card or driver's license). Do not use tweezers.
2. Wash the area with soap and water.
3. Apply ice or a cold pack over the area **Figure 15-5** .
4. Applying a hydrocortisone cream can help combat local swelling and itching. An antihistamine (such as Benadryl) reduces some itching if given early and should be taken as soon as possible. However when taken by mouth, an antihistamine may work too slowly to counteract a life-threatening allergic reaction.
5. Observe the victim for signs of a severe allergic reaction. For a person having a severe allergic reaction, call 9-1-1. If the victim has a prescribed auto-injector, help the victim use it.

▶ Spider Bites

Most spiders are venomous. However, most spiders lack an effective delivery system—long fangs and strong jaws—to bite a human. In North America, death occurs rarely and only from bites by black widow spiders. A spider bite is difficult to diagnose, especially when the spider was not seen or recovered, because the bites typically cause little immediate pain.

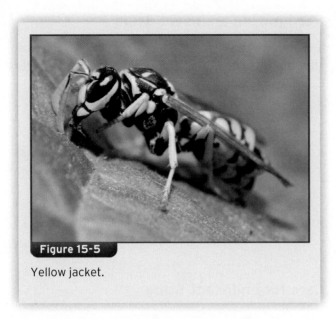

Figure 15-5

Yellow jacket.

Recognizing a Black Widow Spider Bite

Black widow spiders have round abdomens that vary from gray to brown to black, depending on the species. The female black widow often has a shiny black abdomen with a red or yellow spot, often in the shape of an hourglass **Figure 15-6**.

Signs of a black widow spider bite can include the following:

- The victim may feel a sharp pinprick when the spider bites, but some victims are not aware of the bite. Within 15 minutes, a dull, numbing pain develops in the bite area.
- Two small fang marks might be seen as tiny red spots.
- Severe abdominal pain develops (a bite on an arm can cause severe chest pain, mimicking a heart attack).
- Headache, chills, fever, heavy sweating, dizziness, nausea, and vomiting appear next.

Recognizing a Brown Recluse Spider Bite

Brown recluse spiders are also known in North America as fiddle-back and violin spiders. They have a violin-shaped figure on their backs (several other spider species have a similar configuration on their backs). Color varies from fawn to dark brown, with darker legs **Figure 15-7**.

Brown recluse spiders are found primarily in the southern and midwestern states, with other less toxic but related spiders found throughout the rest of the country. They are absent from the Pacific Northwest, where the aggressive house spider, also known as the hobo spider, is found and causes injuries similar to those of the brown recluse.

Signs of a brown recluse and hobo spider bite include the following:

- A local reaction usually occurs within several hours, with mild to severe pain and itching.
- A blister often develops several days later, becomes red, and bursts. During the early stages, the affected area often takes on a bull's-eye appearance, with a central white area surrounded by a reddened area, ringed by a whitish or blue border **Figure 15-8**.
- A scab will form that falls off in a few days, leaving a large ulcer. This process of slow tissue destruction can continue for weeks or months. The ulcer sometimes requires skin grafting.
- Other signs can include headache, fever, weakness, nausea, and vomiting.

Recognizing a Tarantula Spider Bite

Tarantulas bite only when provoked or roughly handled. The bite varies from almost painless to a deep throbbing pain that lasts up to 1 hour.

Care for All Spider Bites

To care for any spider bite:

1. If possible, catch the spider to confirm its identity.
2. Wash the bitten area with soap and water.
3. Apply ice or a cold pack over the bite to relieve pain.
4. Seek medical care. For black widow spider bites, an antivenin exists that can provide relief within a few hours. Small children and frail elderly people are most at risk for severe complications or death.

▶ Scorpion Stings

Scorpions look like miniature lobsters, with lobster-like pincers and a long upcurved "tail" with a poisonous stinger **Figure 15-9**. Several species of scorpions inhabit the southwestern United States, but only the bark scorpion of Arizona is potentially deadly. Small children and frail elderly people are most at risk for severe complications or death.

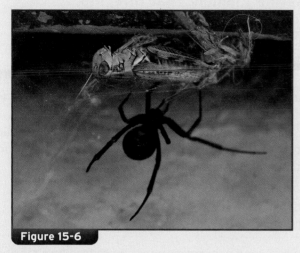

Figure 15-6

Black widow spider. Note red hourglass configuration on abdomen.

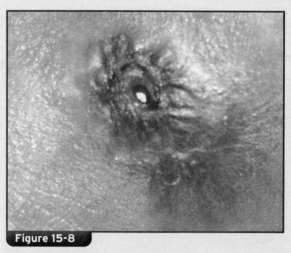

Figure 15-8

Brown recluse spider bite. Note bull's-eye appearance.

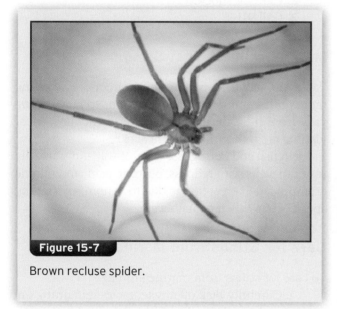

Figure 15-7

Brown recluse spider.

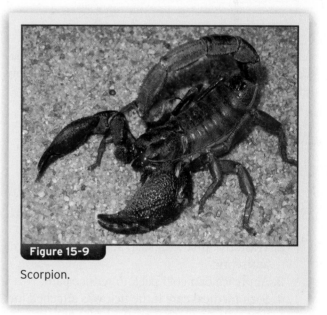

Figure 15-9

Scorpion.

Recognizing a Scorpion Sting

The most frequent sign of a scorpion sting, especially in an adult victim, is local, immediate pain and burning around the sting site. Later, numbness or tingling occurs.

Care for a Scorpion Sting

To care for a scorpion sting:
1. Gently wash the sting site with soap and water or rubbing alcohol.
2. Apply ice or a cold pack over the area.
3. Seek medical care.

▶ Tick Bites

Most tick bites are harmless, although ticks can carry serious diseases **Figure 15-10**. If a tick is carrying a disease, the longer it stays embedded, the greater the chance of disease being transmitted. Because its bite is painless, a tick can remain embedded for days without the victim realizing it.

Two types of ticks can transmit diseases. Deer ticks are small, about the size of the head of a pin. Wood ticks are larger, usually about one quarter of an inch. Depending on where the victim lives, doctors may prescribe preventative treatment for certain

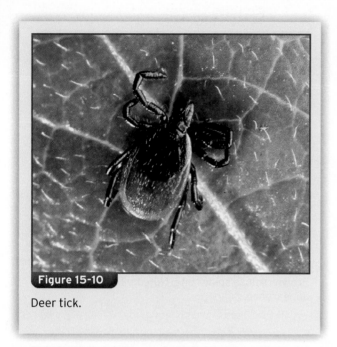

Figure 15-10

Deer tick.

diseases. If a tick is found embedded in a victim, especially if it may have been there for more than a few hours, the victim should seek medical care.

Care for Tick Bites

1. Remove the tick with tweezers or a specialized tick-removal tool. Grasp the tick as close to the skin as possible and lift the tick with enough force to "tent" the skin surface. Hold it in this position until the tick lets go.
2. Wash the area with soap and water or use an antiseptic.
3. Apply ice or a cold pack to reduce pain.
4. Seek medical care if the tick was attached for more than a few hours. If a rash appears, seek medical care. Watch for other signs of disease transmitted by ticks, such as fever, muscle or joint aches, and weakness, and seek medical care if signs develop.

▶ Marine Animal Injuries

Most marine animals bite or sting in defense, rather than attacking. Injuries can include wounds and allergic reactions.

Marine Animals That Bite, Rip, or Puncture

Shark bites are rare and wounds are similar to injuries caused by boat propellers and chain saws.

Barracudas have an undeserved reputation as attackers of humans. The risk of a barracuda bite is exceedingly small.

Moray eels are known to bite divers who handle or tease them, usually in competition for food or in pursuit of lobsters.

Care for Bites, Rips, or Punctures from Marine Animals

To care for a bite, rip, or puncture caused by a marine animal:
1. Control bleeding.
2. Care for shock.
3. Call 9-1-1.

Marine Animals That Sting

Each year, jellyfish and Portuguese man-of-wars sting more than 1 million people. Reactions to being stung vary from mild dermatitis to severe reactions. Most victims recover without medical care.

Jellyfish and Portuguese man-of-war stings usually result in welts with redness, burning pain, and muscle cramping. This reaction is due to venom injected by special cells called nematocysts.

Care for Stings from Marine Animals

To care for stings from marine animals:
1. Carefully pick off any tentacles remaining on the skin. Use gloves if available.
2. Apply vinegar to jellyfish stings for at least 30 seconds to neutralize nematocysts. If vinegar is not available, apply baking soda paste.
3. Immerse the affected part in hot water as soon as possible for at least 25 minutes.
4. Seek medical care.

CAUTION

DO NOT try to rub the tentacles off of the victim's skin; rubbing activates the stinging cells.

Marine Animals That Puncture by Spines

Stingrays, commonly found in tropical and subtropical waters, are peaceful, reclusive bottom feeders that generally lie buried in the sand or mud. Most wounds inflicted by stingrays are produced on the ankle or foot when the victim steps on a ray. The sting is usually more like a laceration because the large tail barb can do significant damage. The venom causes intense burning pain at the site.

Care for Punctures from Marine Animal Spines

To care for punctures from marine animal spines:

1. Relieve pain by immersing the injured body part in hot water for 30 to 90 minutes (hot water helps to neutralize the venom).
2. Wash the wound with soap and water.
3. Flush the area with water under pressure to wash out as much of the toxin and foreign material as possible.
4. Seek medical care.

▶ Emergency Care Wrap-Up

Condition	What to Look For	What to Do
Animal and human bites	• Torn tissue • Bleeding	1. Wash wound with soap and water under pressure. 2. Flush wound thoroughly. 3. Control bleeding. 4. Seek medical care.
Poisonous snake bites	• Severe, burning pain • Small puncture wounds • Swelling • Nausea, vomiting, sweating, weakness • Discoloration and blood-filled blisters developing hours after the bite	1. Get away from the snake. 2. Limit victim's movement. Immobilize the affected limb. 3. Gently wash area with soap and water. 4. For a coral snake bite, apply mild pressure by wrapping the entire affected arm or leg with an elastic bandage. 5. Seek medical care.
Insect stings	• Pain • Itching • Swelling • Severe allergic reaction, including breathing problems	1. Scrape away any stinger. 2. Wash with soap and water. 3. Apply ice or a cold pack. 4. Give hydrocortisone cream and an antihistamine. 5. Observe for signs of a severe allergic reaction. Call 9-1-1 if a severe allergic reaction occurs. If victim has an epinephrine auto-injector, help victim use it.
Spider bites	**Black widow** • May feel sharp pain • Two small fang marks • Severe abdominal pain • Headache, chills, fever, sweating, dizziness, nausea **Brown recluse and hobo** • Blister developing several days later • Ulcer in skin • Headache, fever, weakness, nausea	1. Identify the spider if possible. 2. Wash bitten area with soap and water. 3. Apply ice or a cold pack. 4. Seek medical care.
Scorpion stings	• Pain and burning at sting site • Later, numbness or tingling	1. Wash sting site with soap and water. 2. Apply ice or a cold pack. 3. Seek medical care.
Tick bites	• Tick still attached • Rash (especially one shaped like a bull's-eye) • Fever, joint aches, weakness	1. Remove tick. 2. Wash bitten area with soap and water or use an antiseptic. 3. Apply ice or a cold pack. 4. Seek medical care if the tick was attached for more than a few hours. Seek medical care if rash or other signs such as fever or muscle or joint aches appear.

Condition	What to Look For	What to Do
Marine animal injuries	• Bites, rips, or punctures from marine animals (for example, sharks, barracudas, moray eels)	1. Control bleeding. 2. Care for shock. 3. Call 9-1-1.
	• Stings from marine animals (for example, jellyfish, Portuguese man-of-war)	1. Pick off tentacles. 2. Apply vinegar to jellyfish stings. 3. Immerse the affected part in hot water. 4. Seek medical care.
	• Punctures from marine animal spines (for example, stingray)	1. Immerse injured part in hot water for 30 to 90 minutes. 2. Wash with soap and water. 3. Flush with water under pressure. 4. Seek medical care.

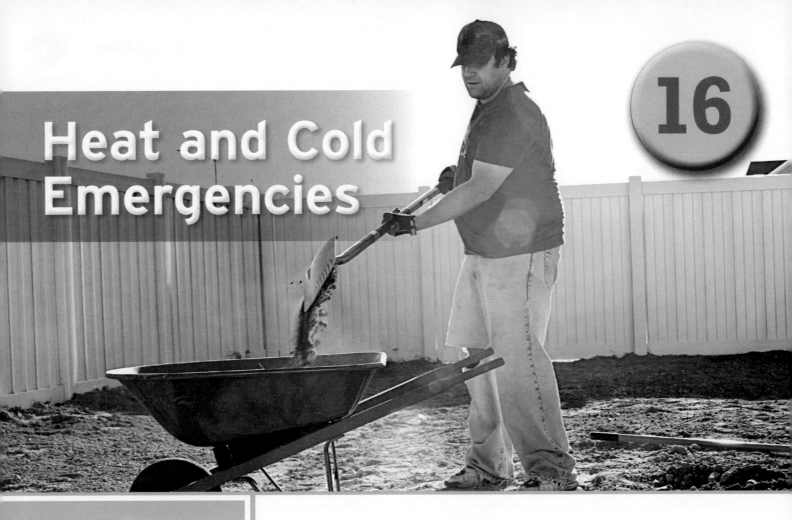

Heat and Cold Emergencies

16

Meeting ⊙SHA Recommendations

This chapter and the accompanying lesson cover the following *OSHA Best Practices Guide: Fundamentals of a Workplace First-Aid Program (2006)*:

5. Responding to Non-Life-Threatening Emergencies

- Temperature extremes
  - Exposure to cold, including frostbite and hypothermia;
  - Exposure to heat, including heat cramps, heat exhaustion and heatstroke.

▶ Heat Emergencies

Prolonged exposure to high temperatures or physical activity in a hot environment can cause these heat-related illnesses: heat cramps, heat exhaustion, and heatstroke.

Recognizing Heat Cramps

> **heat cramps**
> Painful muscle spasms, often in the legs.

Heat cramps are painful muscle spasms that occur suddenly, often after physical exertion. They usually involve the muscles in the back of the leg (calf and hamstring muscles) but may also involve the abdomen.

Care for Heat Cramps

To care for heat cramps:
1. Have the victim stop activity and rest in a cool area.
2. Stretch the cramped muscle.
3. If the victim is responsive and not nauseated, provide water or a commercial sports drink (such as Gatorade® or Powerade®).

Recognizing Heat Exhaustion

> **heat exhaustion**
> Condition caused by the loss of the body's water and salt through excessive sweating.

Heat exhaustion is caused by the loss of water and salt through heavy sweating. Heat exhaustion affects those who do not drink enough fluid while working or exercising in hot environments and those not acclimated to hot, humid conditions.

The signs of heat exhaustion can include the following:

- Heavy sweating
- Severe thirst
- Weakness
- Headache
- Nausea and vomiting

Care for Heat Exhaustion

To care for heat exhaustion:

1. Have the victim stop activity and rest in a cool area.
2. Remove any excess or tight clothing.
3. If the victim is responsive and not nauseated, provide water or a commercial sports drink.
4. Have the victim lie down.
5. Apply cool packs to the armpits and to the crease where the legs attach to the pelvis.
6. Seek medical care if the condition does not improve within 30 minutes. Children or frail adults should be seen by a medical professional.

CAUTION

DO NOT place the victim in an ice bath.
DO NOT cool the victim so much that the victim begins to shiver.

Recognizing Heatstroke

heatstroke
Condition in which the body's heat-regulating ability becomes overwhelmed and ceases to function properly, resulting in an inability to sweat and a dangerously high body temperature.

Heatstroke is a life-threatening condition in which the body becomes dangerously overheated. Heatstroke can occur quickly (for example, to a long-distance runner during a very hot day) or it can take days to develop (for example, to an elderly person without air conditioning during a heat wave).

The signs of heatstroke can include the following:

- Extremely hot skin
- Dry skin (may be wet from strenuous work or exercise)
- Confusion
- Seizures
- Unresponsiveness

Care for Heatstroke

To care for heatstroke:

1. Call 9-1-1.
2. Cool the victim immediately by whatever means possible: cool, wet towels or sheets to the head and body accompanied by fanning, and/or cold packs against the armpits, sides of neck, and groin.
3. If unresponsive and not breathing, start CPR.

▶ Cold Emergencies

When exposed to very cold environments, the body may become overwhelmed. Cold exposure may cause injury to parts of the body (frostbite) or to the body as a whole (hypothermia).

Frostbite

Frostbite happens only when temperatures drop below freezing. It affects mainly the feet, hands, ears, and nose **Figures 16-1A, B**. When skin tissue dies (gangrene) from frostbite, an affected part may have to be amputated.

frostbite
Tissue damage caused by extreme cold.

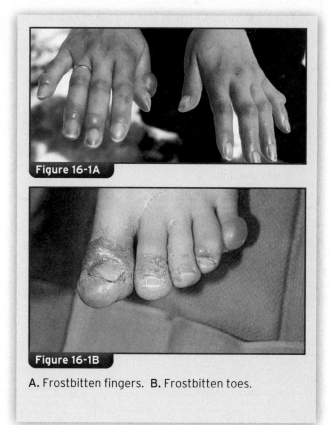

Figure 16-1A

Figure 16-1B

A. Frostbitten fingers. **B.** Frostbitten toes.

The signs of frostbite include the following:
- White, waxy-looking skin
- Skin feels cold and numb (pain at first, followed by numbness)
- Blisters, which may appear after rewarming

Care for Frostbite

To care for frostbite:
1. Move the victim to a warm place.
2. Remove wet/cold clothing and jewelry from the injured part.
3. Seek medical care.

CAUTION

DO NOT rub or massage the frostbitten area.

FYI

Caring for Frostbite in a Remote Location

If the victim is in a remote location (more than 1 hour from medical care) and you have warm water, use the following rewarming method:

1. Place the frostbitten part in warm (100°F) water for 20 to 40 minutes or until the tissue becomes soft. For ear or facial injuries, apply warm, moist cloths and change them frequently.

2. After thawing:
   - Place dry dressings between fingers or toes.
   - Slightly elevate the affected part to reduce pain and swelling.
   - Provide ibuprofen or acetaminophen for pain and swelling.

hypothermia
A dangerous condition caused by severe exposure to cold in which the core body temperature drops below 95°F.

Recognizing Hypothermia

Hypothermia develops when the body's temperature drops to about 95°F.

Hypothermia can develop either quickly (for example, cold water immersion) or gradually during prolonged exposure to a cold environment. The temperature does not have to be below freezing for hypothermia to occur.

The signs of hypothermia include the following:
- Uncontrollable shivering
- Confusion, sluggishness
- Cold skin even under clothing

Care for Hypothermia

To care for hypothermia:
1. Get the victim out of the cold.
2. Prevent heat loss by:
   - Replacing wet clothing with dry clothing
   - Covering the victim's head
   - Placing insulation (such as blankets, towels, coats) beneath and over the victim
3. Have the victim rest in a comfortable position.
4. If the victim is alert and able to swallow, give him or her warm, sugary beverages.
5. Seek medical care for severe hypothermia (rigid muscles, cold skin on abdomen, confusion, lethargy).

FYI

An Ounce of Prevention

Prepare appropriately for any environment.

For a hot environment:
- Wear lightweight, loose-fitting clothes and a hat with a wide brim.
- Drink adequate water or commercial sports drinks.
- Take breaks in cooler areas.

For a cold environment:
- Layer clothing, with moisture-wicking clothing near the skin and outer layers that are windproof and waterproof but breathable material.
- Keep head and neck covered to minimize heat loss.
- Drink warm drinks and eat properly.

▶ Emergency Care Wrap-Up

Condition	What to Look For	What to Do
Heat cramps	• Painful muscle spasm during or after physical activity • Usually lower leg affected	1. Move victim to cool place. 2. Stretch the cramped muscle. 3. If the victim is responsive, give water or sports drink.
Heat exhaustion	• Heavy sweating • Severe thirst • Weakness • Headache • Nausea and vomiting	1. Move victim to cool place. 2. Have victim lie down. 3. Apply cool packs to the armpits and the crease where the legs attach to the pelvis. 4. If victim is responsive, give water or sports drink. 5. Seek medical care if no improvement within 30 minutes.
Heatstroke	• Extremely hot skin • Dry skin (may be wet at first) • Confusion • Seizures • Unresponsiveness	1. Call 9-1-1. 2. Cool the victim immediately by whatever means possible: cool, wet towels or sheets to the head and body accompanied by fanning, and/or cold packs against the armpits, sides of neck, and groin. 3. If unresponsive and not breathing, start CPR.
Frostbite	• White, waxy-looking skin • Skin feels cold and numb (pain at first, followed by numbness) • Blisters, which may appear after rewarming	1. Move victim to warm place. 2. Remove wet/cold clothing and jewelry from injured part(s). 3. Seek medical care.

Hypothermia	**Mild**
	• Uncontrollable shivering
	• Confusion, sluggishness
	• Cold skin even under clothing
	
	Severe
	• No shivering
	• Muscles stiff and rigid
	• Skin ice cold
	• Appears to be dead
		1. Move victim to warm place.
		2. Prevent heat loss by
		  • Replacing wet clothing with dry clothing
		  • Covering victim's head
		3. Have victim lie down.
		4. Give warm, sugary beverages if alert and sitting up.
		5. Seek medical care if needed.

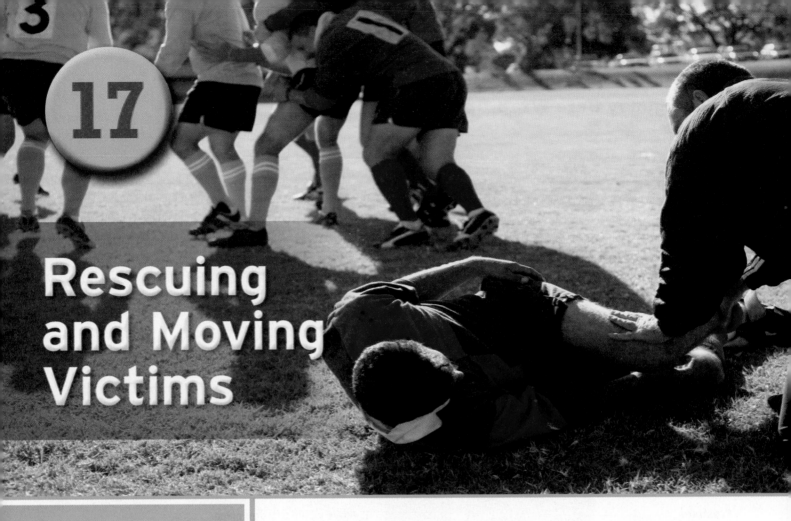

17

Rescuing and Moving Victims

Meeting ⊙SHA Recommendations

This chapter and the accompanying lesson cover the following *OSHA Best Practices Guide: Fundamentals of a Workplace First-Aid Program (2006)*:

3. Assessing the Scene and the Victim(s)

- Assessing the toxic potential of the environment and the need for respiratory protection;

- Establishing the presence of a confined space and the need for respiratory protection and specialized training to perform a rescue;

- Prioritizing care when there are several injured;

- Indications for and methods of safety moving and rescuing victim(s);

- Repositioning ill/injured victims to prevent further injury.

(continues on next page)

▶ Water Rescue

"Reach-throw-row-go" identifies the sequence for attempting a water rescue:

- If the victim is within reach and you are securely anchored, extend your arm or an object such as a pole or long stick.
- If the victim is slightly farther away, throw anything that floats (such as a life jacket or throw line).
- If the victim is out of throwing range and there is a boat (such as a canoe, kayak, or rowboat), row to the victim. You could also paddle to the victim using a surfboard or boogie board, or use a motorized water craft if available. Wear a personal flotation device (PFD) for your own safety.
- If none of these procedures is possible and you are trained in water lifesaving procedures, you might swim to the victim.

> **CAUTION**
>
> **DO NOT** swim to and grasp a drowning person unless you are trained to make the rescue.

Meeting OSHA Recommendations

4. Responding to Life-Threatening Emergencies
- Inhaled poisons: carbon monoxide; hydrogen sulfide; smoke; and other chemical fumes, vapors, and gases;
- Recognizing asphyxiation and the danger of entering a confined space without appropriate respiratory protection.

► Ice Rescue

If a person has fallen through the ice near the shore:
- Extend a pole or throw a line with a floatable object attached to it. When the person has hold of the object, pull him or her toward the shore or the edge of the ice.

► Electrical Emergency Rescue

- Most indoor electrocutions are caused by faulty electrical equipment or careless use of electrical appliances. Before you touch the victim, turn off the electricity at the circuit breaker, fuse box, or outside switch box.
- If the electrocution involves high-voltage power lines, the power must be turned off before anyone approaches the victim. Wait for trained personnel with the proper equipment to cut the wires or disconnect them.
- If a power line has fallen over a car, tell the driver and passengers to stay still in the car. A victim should attempt to jump out of the car only if an explosion or fire threatens his or her life. The victim must not make contact with the car or the wire and the ground at the same time.
- Do not approach a victim in a pool or puddle of water containing a downed power line. The water can conduct electricity.

► Hazardous Materials Incidents

Almost any highway crash scene involves the potential danger of hazardous chemicals. Clues that indicate the presence of hazardous materials include signs on vehicles (for example, Explosive, Flammable, or Corrosive), spilled liquids or solids, strong, unusual odors, and clouds of vapor **Figure 17-1**. Stay well away and upwind from the area. Only people who are specially trained in handling hazardous materials and who have the proper equipment should be in the area.

► Motor Vehicle Crashes

1. Stop and park your vehicle in a safe area. Call 9-1-1.
2. Turn on your vehicle's emergency hazard flashers. Raise the hood of your vehicle to draw more attention to the scene.

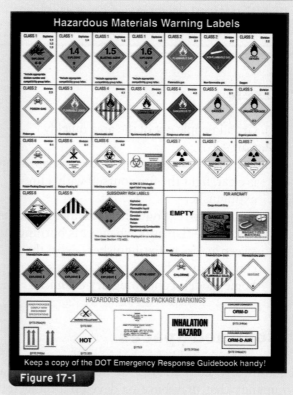

Figure 17-1

Hazardous materials warning signs.

3. Make sure that the scene is safe before approaching the crash.
4. Ask the driver(s) to turn off the ignition of the involved car(s), or turn it off yourself.
5. Place flares or reflectors 250 to 500 feet behind the crash scene to warn oncoming drivers of the crash. Do not ignite flares around leaking gasoline or diesel fuel.
6. If you suspect a victim has a spinal injury, use your hands to stabilize the person's head and neck.
7. Check and care for any life-threatening injuries first, and then handle lesser injuries.

CAUTION

DO NOT rush to get victims out of a car that has been in a crash. Most vehicle crashes do not involve fire, and most vehicles stay in an upright position.

DO NOT move or allow victims to move unless there is an immediate danger, such as fire or oncoming traffic.

DO NOT transport victims in your car or any other bystander's vehicle.

▶ Fires

1. Get all people out of the area quickly.
2. Call 9-1-1.
3. If the fire is small and your own escape route is clear, fight the fire yourself with a fire extinguisher.
4. To use a fire extinguisher, aim directly at the base of the flames of whatever is burning and sweep across it. Extinguishers expel their contents quickly: in 8 to 25 seconds for most home models containing dry chemicals.

▶ Confined Spaces

A confined space is an area not intended for human occupancy that may have or develop a dangerous atmosphere. Below-ground confined spaces include manholes, utility vaults, storage tanks, old mines, and wells. Ground-level confined spaces include industrial tanks and farm storage silos. Above-ground confined spaces include water towers and storage tanks.

An emergency in a confined space demands immediate action. If someone enters a confined space and signals for help or becomes unresponsive, follow these steps:

1. Call 9-1-1.
2. Check motionless victims first. Do not enter the confined space unless you have the proper training and equipment, such as a self-contained air supply, safety harness, and lifeline.
3. Once the victim is removed, provide care.

▶ Triage: What to Do With Multiple Victims

You may encounter emergency situations in which there is more than one victim. If the scene is safe, decide who must be cared for first. This process of prioritizing or classifying multiple victims is called **triage**.

triage
The sorting of patients into groups according to the severity of injuries. Used to determine priorities for treatment and transport.

To find those needing immediate care for life-threatening conditions, ask all victims who can get up and walk to move to a specific area. Victims who can get up and walk rarely have life-threatening injuries. These victims are known as the "walking wounded." Do not force a victim to move if he or she reports pain.

It is important to determine who needs life-saving treatment immediately. Check motionless victims first, since they will generally be in more serious condition than those who are able to move. Check for breathing. If the victim is not breathing, open the airway and, if possible, place the victim in the recovery position. Check for severe, life-threatening bleeding and provide care, if possible. Enlist bystanders to assist by applying direct pressure to any bleeding or to maintain an open airway. Rapidly move to the next victim. Spend no more than 30 seconds with each victim. Once you have tended to the needs of the most severely injured, go back and reassess for less serious injuries. You will usually be relieved of your responsibilities when EMS arrives on the scene.

Classify victims according to the following care and transportation priorities:

1. *Immediate care:* Victim needs immediate care and transport to medical care as soon as possible.
   - Breathing difficulties
   - Severe bleeding
   - Severe burns
   - Signs of shock
   - Unresponsiveness
2. *Delayed care:* Care and transportation can be delayed up to 1 hour.
   - Minor extremity burns
   - Bone or joint injuries without significant bleeding
   - Back injuries with or without suspected spinal cord damage unless difficulty of breathing is present
3. *Walking wounded:* Care and transportation can be delayed up to 3 hours.
   - Minor fractures
   - Minor wounds
4. *Dead:* Victim is obviously dead or unlikely to survive because of the type or extent of injuries.

▶ Moving Victims

A victim should not be moved until he or she is ready for transportation to a hospital, if required. A victim should be moved only if there is an immediate danger, such as the following:

- Fire or danger of fire
- Explosives or other hazardous materials
- Impossible to protect the scene from hazards
- Impossible to gain access to other victims in the situation who need lifesaving care (such as in a motor vehicle crash)

Emergency Moves

The major danger in moving a victim quickly is the possibility of aggravating an injury. For a victim lying on the ground, pull the victim in the direction of the long axis of the body to provide as much protection

to the spinal cord as possible. Several methods exist for moving victims:

Drags:
- *Shoulder drag:* Use for short distances over a rough surface; stabilize victim's head with your forearms Figure 17-2 .
- *Ankle drag:* This is the fastest method for a short distance on a smooth surface Figure 17-3 .
- *Blanket pull:* Roll the victim onto a blanket and pull from behind the victim's head Figure 17-4 .

One-person moves:
- *Human crutch (one person helps victim walk):* If one leg is injured, help the victim walk on the good leg while you support the injured side Figure 17-5 .
- *Cradle carry:* Use this method for children and lightweight adults who cannot walk Figure 17-6 .
- *Fire fighter's carry:* If the victim's injuries permit, you can travel longer distances if you carry the victim over your shoulder Figure 17-7 .
- *Pack-strap carry:* When injuries make the fire fighter's carry unsafe, this method is better for longer distances Figure 17-8 .
- *Piggyback carry:* Use this method when the victim cannot walk but can use his or her arms to hang onto the rescuer Figure 17-9 .

Two-person or three-person moves:
- *Two-person assist:* This method is similar to the human crutch Figure 17-10 .
- *Two-handed seat carry:* Two people carry the victim Figure 17-11 .
- *Extremity carry:* One person supports the victim underneath the victim's arms while the other person supports the victim's legs Figure 17-12 .

Nonemergency Moves

All injured parts should be stabilized before and during moving. If rapid transportation is not needed, it is helpful to practice on another person about the same size as the injured victim.

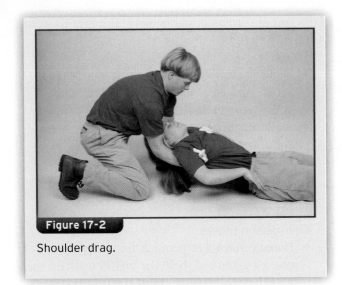

Figure 17-2

Shoulder drag.

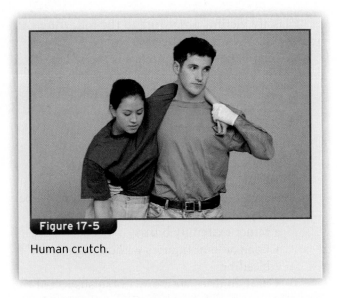

Figure 17-5

Human crutch.

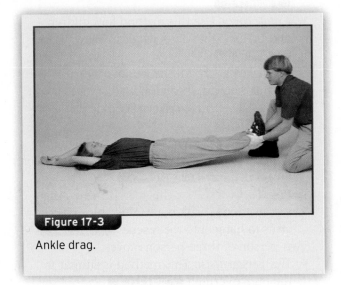

Figure 17-3

Ankle drag.

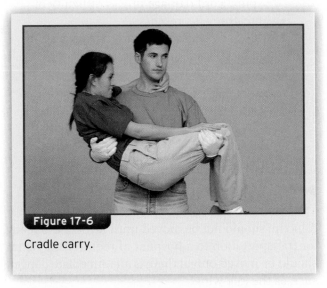

Figure 17-6

Cradle carry.

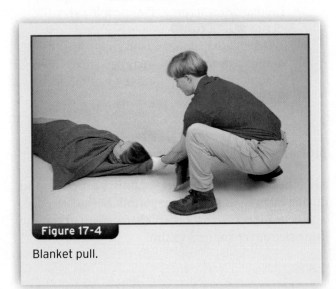

Figure 17-4

Blanket pull.

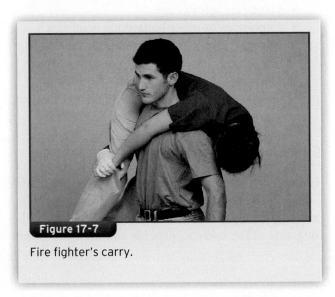

Figure 17-7

Fire fighter's carry.

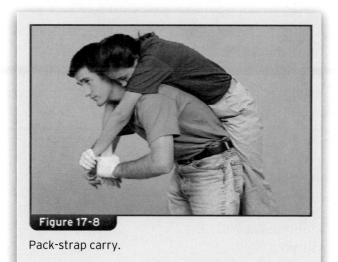

Figure 17-8

Pack-strap carry.

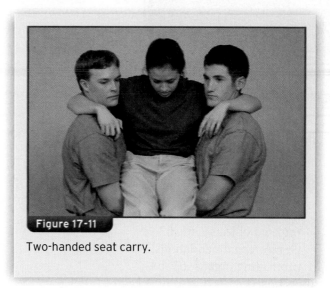

Figure 17-11

Two-handed seat carry.

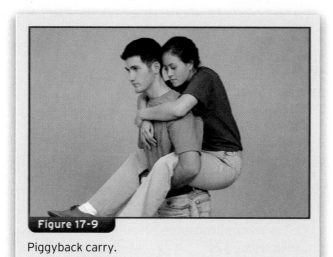

Figure 17-9

Piggyback carry.

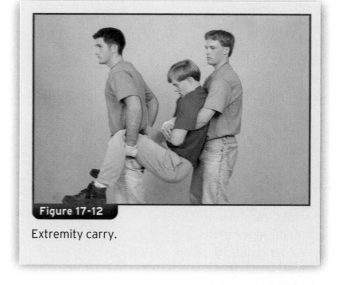

Figure 17-12

Extremity carry.

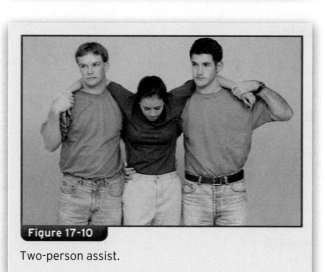

Figure 17-10

Two-person assist.

index

impaled objects
   abdomen, in, 63
   chests, in, 62, 64
   OSHA recommendations, 61
   wound care, 39, 41
implanted devices, and AED
      use, 27, 29
implied consent, defined, 4
incisions, 35, 36
infants
   airway obstruction, 23
   CPR, 16, 17, 21
infected wounds, 38, 41
information, gathering, about injury
      victims, 14
ingested poisons
   care for, 81, 84
   signs of, 80, 84
inhaled poisoning, 80, 82, 84
injuries. *See also specific types of injuries*
   nonfatal, causes of, 1, 2
   not aggravating, 14
insect stings
   anaphylaxis, 85, 87, 92
   care for, 87, 92
   signs of, 87, 92
internal bleeding
   care for, 39–40, 41
   recognizing, 39, 41
iron poisoning, 81

J

jellyfish stings, 90, 93
joint injuries. *See also* splints
   care for, 67–68, 72, 73
   dislocations, 67, 68, 73
   OSHA recommendations, 65
   signs of, 67, 68, 73
   sprains, 67, 73

K

kerosene poisoning, 81

L

lacerations
   eyes, to, 55, 56, 59
   skin, 35

legal issues and first aid, 2–4
lips, bitten, 57, 60

M

marine animal injuries
   bites, rips and punctures, 90, 93
   punctures from spines, 91, 93
   stings, 90, 93
Material Safety Data Sheets (MSDSs)
   chemical burns, 49
   chemical safety at the
      worksite, 82
medical care
   seeking, 6–7
   wounds requiring, 39
medical emergencies
   breathing difficulty, 75–76, 79
   chest pain, 75, 79
   consciousness, changes in, 74–75
   diabetic emergencies, 76–78, 79
   fainting, 76, 79
   OSHA recommendations, 74
   pregnancy emergencies, 78, 79
   seizures, 76, 79
medical identification tags, 14
medications
   expiration dates, 2
   first aid kit, in, 2
   patches, and AED use, 27, 29
   SAMPLE history and, 14
methanol poisoning, 81
mobility, after head injuries, 54
moray eel bites, 90, 93
motor vehicle crashes, 99–100
mouth injuries
   aspiration of blood and/or
      teeth, 52, 58
   bitten lip or tongue, 52, 57, 60
   broken teeth, 52, 58
   knocked-out teeth, 52, 57–58, 60
   toothache, 58, 60
mouth-to-barrier devices, 17
mouth-to-nose method, 17
mouth-to-stoma method, 17
muscle injuries
   care for, 68, 73
   contusions, 65, 68, 73
   cramps, 65, 68, 73
   OSHA recommendations, 65

extent of, 47–48, 51

first-degree, care for, 48, 51

respiratory injury, 48

second degree, large area, and third degree, care
for, 49, 51

second degree, small area, care for, 48–49, 51

third-degree (full-thickness) burns, 46, 47, 51

tick bites

care for, 90, 92

dangerous types, 89–90

signs of, 92

tongue

airway obstruction, 18

bitten, 57, 60

triage

defined, 100

performing, 100–101

tuberculosis (TB), 7

Twinject, 44

two-handed seat carry, 101, 103

two-person assist, 101, 103

V

venous bleeding, 34, 35

ventricular fibrillation (V-fib), 26

ventricular tachycardia (V-tach), 26

victims, moving

emergency moves, 101, 102–103

nonemergency moves, 101

victims, rescuing

confined spaces, 100

electrical emergency rescue, 99

fires, 100

hazardous materials incidents, 99

ice rescue, 99

motor vehicle crashes, 99–100

OSHA recommendations, 98–99

triage, 100–101

water rescue, 98

vision problems, after head injuries, 54

vomiting

head injuries, 54

shock, 43

W

walking wounded, classifying
victims as, 101

water

AED use, 27, 29

burns, 48, 49

water moccasin snakes, 86

water rescue, 98

wheezing, 11

wood ticks, 89–90

wounds

amputations, 35, 36, 38, 41

cleaning, 35–36

dressings and bandages, 36, 37, 40

impaled objects, 39, 41

minor wounds, 41

open, checking for, 11

OSHA recommendations, 34

sutures, 40

types of injuries, 35, 36

wound infection, 38, 41

wounds requiring medical care, 39

image credits

Chapter 1
Opener © Corbis/age fotostock; **1-1** Source: U.S. Dept. of Labor; **1-3** Courtesy of Ellis and Associates.

Chapter 3
Opener © Ingram Publishing/age fotostock; **3-4** © Jonathan Noden-Wilkinson/ShutterStock, Inc.; **3-13** © LiquidLibrary

Chapter 4
Opener © Berta A. Daniels, 2010; **4-2** © Berta A. Daniels, 2010; **Skill Drill 4-1** © Berta A. Daniels, 2010

Chapter 5
Opener © Berta A. Daniels, 2010; **5-3, 5-4, 5-5** From *Arrhythmia Recognition: The Art of Interpretation*, courtesy of Tomas B. Garcia, MD.; **5-8** Courtesy of Phillips Medical Systems. All rights reserved.

Chapter 6
Opener © mangostock/ShutterStock, Inc.

Chapter 7
7-2B © English/Custom Medical Stock Photo; **7-2D** © E. M. Singletary, M.D. Used with permission.

Chapter 8
8-2 Courtesy of Dey, L.P.

Chapter 9
Opener © Scott Camazine/Photo Researchers, Inc.; **9-1** © Amy Walters/ShutterStock, Inc.; **9-2** © E. M. Singletary, M.D. Used with permission.; **9-9** © Chuck Stewart, MD.

Chapter 10
Opener © Joe Gough/ShutterStock, Inc.

Chapter 11
Opener © Gordon Swanson/ShutterStock, Inc.

Chapter 12
Opener © Christoph & Friends/Das Fotoarchiv/Alamy Images; **12-2** © E. M. Singletary, M.D. Used with permission.; **Skill Drill 12-4** © Berta A. Daniels, 2010

Chapter 13
Opener © Kzenon/ShutterStock, Inc.

Chapter 14
14-2A © Thomas Photography LLC/Alamy Images; **14-2B** © Thomas J. Peterson/Alamy Images; **14-2C** Courtesy of U.S. Fish & Wildlife Service

Chapter 15
Opener © Jonathan Plant/Alamy Images; **15-1** © Chuck Stewart, MD.; **15-2** © Amee Cross/ShutterStock, Inc.; **15-5** © Arlindo Ferreira da Silva/ShutterStock, Inc.; **15-6** © Crystal Kirk/ShutterStock, Inc.; **15-7** Courtesy of Kenneth Cramer, Monmouth College; **15-8** Courtesy of Department of Entomology, University of Nebraska; **15-9** © Kirubeshwaran/ShutterStock, Inc.; **15-10** Courtesy of Scott Bauer/USDA

Chapter 16
Opener © Yobro10/Dreamstime.com; **16-1A** Courtesy of Neil Malcom Winkelmann

Chapter 17
17-1 Courtesy of the U.S. Department of Transportation